INTERVENTIONAL CARDIOLOGY CLINICS

www.interventional.theclinics.com

Editor-in-Chief

MARVIN H. ENG

Special Topics in Interventional Cardiology

July 2022 • Volume 11 • Number 3

Editor

MARVIN H. ENG

ELSEVIER

1600 John F. Kennedy Boulevard • Suite 1800 • Philadelphia, Pennsylvania, 19103-2899

http://www.theclinics.com

INTERVENTIONAL CARDIOLOGY CLINICS Volume 11, Number 3
July 2022 ISSN 2211-7458, ISBN-13: 978-0-323-84991-3

Editor: Joanna Collett
Developmental Editor: Arlene B. Campos

Interventional Cardiology Clinics (ISSN 2211-7458) is published quarterly by Elsevier Inc., 360 Park Avenue South, New York, NY 10010-1710. Months of issue are January, April, July, and October. Subscription prices are USD 209 per year for US individuals, USD 641 for US institutions, USD 100 per year for US students, USD 209 per year for Canadian individuals, USD 660 for Canadian institutions, USD 100 per year for Canadian students, USD 296 per year for international individuals, USD 660 for international institutions, and USD 150 per year for international students. To receive student/resident rate, orders must be accompanied by name of affiliated institution, date of term, and the *signature* of program/residency coordinator on institution letterhead. Orders will be billed at individual rate until proof of status is received. Foreign air speed delivery is included in all *Clinics* subscription prices. All prices are subject to change without notice. **POSTMASTER:** Send address changes to *Interventional Cardiology Clinics*, Elsevier Health Sciences Division, Subscription Customer Service, 3251 Riverport Lane, Maryland Heights, MO 63043. **Customer Service: Telephone: 1-800-654-2452** (U.S. and Canada); **1-314-447-8871** (outside U.S. and Canada). **Fax: 1-314-447-8029. E-mail: journalscustomerservice-usa@elsevier.com (for print support); journalsonlinesupport-usa@elsevier.com (for online support).**

Reprints. For copies of 100 or more of articles in this publication, please contact the Commercial Reprints Department, Elsevier Inc., 360 Park Avenue South, New York, NY 10010-1710. Tel.: 212-633-3874; Fax: 212-633-3820; E-mail: reprints@elsevier.com.

CONTRIBUTORS

EDITOR-IN-CHIEF

MARVIN H. ENG, MD
Structural Heart Program Medical Director,
Structural Heart Disease Fellowship Director,

AUTHORS

VIKAS AGGARWAL, MD, MPH
Division of Cardiology (Frankel Cardiovascular
Center), Department of Internal Medicine,
University of Michigan Medical School, Ann
Arbor, Michigan, USA

OWAIS KHADEM ALSROUJI, MBBS
Department of Neurosurgery, Henry Ford
Hospital, Detroit, Michigan, USA

VASILIS C. BABALIAROS, MD
Structural Heart and Valve Center, Emory
University Hospital, Atlanta, Georgia, USA

CHRISTOPHER G. BRUCE, MB ChB
Cardiovascular Branch, Division of Intramural
Research, National Heart Lung and Blood
Institute, National Institutes of Health,
Bethesda, Maryland, USA

ARKA CHATTERJEE, MD
Associate Professor of Medicine, Section of
Cardiology, Department of Internal Medicine,
Banner University Medical Center, Sarver
Heart Center, Tucson, Arizona, USA

SAURAV CHATTERJEE, MD
Division of Cardiovascular Medicine, North
Shore-Long Island Jewish Medical Centers,
Northwell Health, Donald and Barbara Zucker
School of Medicine at Hofstra/Northwell, New
York, New York, USA

ALEX BOU CHEBL, MD, FSVIN
Director, Division of Vascular Neurology,
Department of Neurology, Director, Harris
Comprehensive Stroke Center, Henry Ford
Health System, Detroit, Michigan, USA

MARVIN H. ENG, MD
Division of Cardiology, Medical Director,
Structural Heart Program, Structural Heart

Director of Cardiovascular Quality, Banner
University Medical Center, Phoenix, Arizona,
USA

Fellowship Director, Director of
Cardiovascular Quality, Associate Professor of
Medicine, University of Arizona, Banner
University Medical Center, Phoenix, Arizona,
USA

KENITH FANG, MD
Division of Cardiothoracic Surgery, Banner
University Medical Center, Phoenix, Arizona,
USA

ROBERT FRASER, MD
Center for Valve and Structural Heart Disease,
Minneapolis Heart Institute at Abbott
Northwestern Hospital, Hypertrophic
Cardiomyopathy Center, Minneapolis Heart
Institute Foundation, Minneapolis, Minnesota,
USA

MARAT FUDIM, MD, MHS
Division of Cardiology, Duke University
Medical Center, Duke Clinical Research
Institute, Durham, North Carolina, USA

ISHAN GARG, MBBS
Department of Internal Medicine, University of
New Mexico Health Sciences Center,
Albuquerque, New Mexico, USA

ADAM B. GREENBAUM, MD
Cardiovascular Branch, Division of Intramural
Research, National Heart Lung and Blood
Institute, National Institutes of Health,
Bethesda, Maryland, USA; Emory Structural
Heart and Valve Center, Atlanta, Georgia,
USA

ALEXANDER G. HAJDUCZOK, MD
Department of Cardiology, Thomas Jefferson
University Hospital, Philadelphia,
Pennsylvania, USA

KEVIN M. HARRIS, MD
Center for Valve and Structural Heart Disease, Minneapolis Heart Institute at Abbott Northwestern Hospital, Hypertrophic Cardiomyopathy Center, Minneapolis Heart Institute Foundation, Minneapolis, Minnesota, USA

TIMOTHY D. HENRY, MD, FACC, MSCAI
Medical Director, The Carl and Edyth Lindner Center for Research and Education, The Carl and Edyth Lindner Family Distinguished Chair in Clinical Research, Director of Programmatic and Network Development, The Christ Hospital, Cincinnati, Ohio, USA

S. NABEEL HYDER, MD
Division of Cardiology (Frankel Cardiovascular Center), Department of Internal Medicine, University of Michigan Medical School, Ann Arbor, Michigan, USA

ISHAN KAMAT, MD
Section of Cardiology, Baylor College of Medicine, Houston, Texas, USA

JAFFAR M. KHAN, BM BCh, PhD
Cardiovascular Branch, Division of Intramural Research, National Heart Lung and Blood Institute, National Institutes of Health, Bethesda, Maryland, USA

KWAN LEE, MD
Associate Professor of Medicine, Section of Cardiology, Department of Internal Medicine, Banner University Medical Center, Sarver Heart Center, Tucson, Arizona, USA

REBEKAH LANTZ, DO
The Lindner Research Center at the Christ Hospital, Cincinnati, Ohio, USA

ROBERT J. LEDERMAN, MD
Cardiovascular Branch, Division of Intramural Research, National Heart Lung and Blood Institute, National Institutes of Health, Bethesda, Maryland, USA

PHILIPP LURZ, MD, PhD
Department of Cardiology, Heart Center Leipzig, University of Leipzig, Germany, USA

GEORGIA MATTINGLY, BA
The Lindner Research Center at the Christ Hospital, Cincinnati, Ohio, USA

RYAN C. MAVES, MD, FCCM, FCCP, FIDSA
Departments of Internal Medicine and Anesthesiology, Wake Forest School of Medicine, Winston-Salem, North California, USA

ABDUL MANNAN KHAN MINHAS, MD
Department of Internal Medicine, Forrest General Hospital, Hattiesburg, Mississippi, USA

KESHAV R. NAYAK, MD, FACC, FSCAI
Department of Cardiology, Scripps Mercy Hospital San Diego, San Diego, California, USA

MANESH R. PATEL, MD
Division of Cardiology, Duke University Medical Center, Duke Clinical Research Institute, Durham, North California, USA

ODAYME QUESADA, MD
Director of the Women's Heart Program at The Christ Hospital, Cincinnati, Ohio, USA

TOBY ROGERS, BM BCh, PhD
Cardiovascular Branch, Division of Intramural Research, National Heart Lung and Blood Institute, National Institutes of Health, Bethesda, Maryland, USA; MedStar Washington Hospital Center, Washington, DC, USA

HUSAM SALAH, MD
Department of Medicine, Arkansas Medical University, Arkansas, USA

MADHAN SHANMUGASUNDARAM, MD
Associate Professor of Medicine, Section of Cardiology, Department of Internal Medicine, Banner University Medical Center, Sarver Heart Center, Tucson, Arizona, USA

ABU BAKER SHEIKH, MD
Department of Internal Medicine, University of New Mexico Health Sciences Center, Albuquerque, New Mexico, USA

ASHER A. SOBOTKA
University of Pennsylvania, Philadelphia, Pennsylvania, USA

PAUL A. SOBOTKA, MD
Division of Cardiology, The Ohio State University, Columbus, Ohio, USA

PAUL SORAJJA, MD
Center for Valve and Structural Heart Disease,
Minneapolis Heart Institute at Abbott
Northwestern Hospital, Roger L. and Lynn C.
Headrick Family Chair, Valve Science Center,
Abbott Northwestern Hospital, Hypertrophic
Cardiomyopathy Center, Minneapolis Heart
Institute Foundation, Minneapolis, Minnesota,
USA

ROBERT STEFFEN, MD
Center for Valve and Structural Heart Disease,
Minneapolis Heart Institute at Abbott
Northwestern Hospital, Hypertrophic
Cardiomyopathy Center, Minneapolis Heart
Institute Foundation, Minneapolis, Minnesota,
USA

VARUN TANDON, MD
Division of Cardiology, Banner University
Medical Center, Phoenix, Arizona, USA

CONTENTS

> Paravalvular leaks (PVLs) are challenging lesions that require a comprehensive understanding of surgical and transcatheter heart therapies, multimodality imaging, and transcatheter techniques. Approach to a transcatheter heart valve (THV) or surgical prosthesis for PVL differs in terms of options and varies according to the location (aortic or mitral). A suggested framework for transcatheter PVL repair is defect localization, access planning, defect crossing, sheath delivery. and occluder deployment. Careful planning facilitates success, but operators begin the case with a flexible mindset because many initial strategies may not succeed.

> Over the past several decades, alcohol septal ablation has become an established therapy for selected patients, in whom there is clinical improvement in symptoms as well as objective functional capacity. Patient selection is essential to success, with continued emphasis on the procedure being performed by experienced operators as part of a multidisciplinary team. In many patients, the outcomes of alcohol septal ablation are comparable to the standard of surgical myectomy. The optimization of the outcomes of alcohol septal ablation is essential for the longitudinal care of patients with hypertrophic cardiomyopathy.

> Transcatheter electrosurgery is a versatile tool that can be used to cut cardiac tissue without the need for a sternotomy, cardiopulmonary bypass, and cardioplegia. With adequate imaging and suitable anatomy, any cardiac tissue can be cut. Thus, transcatheter electrosurgery can provide bespoke therapies for complex patients who often have no other good treatment options. In this review, we will discuss the common applications for electrosurgical tissue traversal and laceration, including transcaval access, BASILICA, LAMPOON, and ELASTA-Clip, summarizing the evidence and the key technical steps for each.

Device therapy for severe heart failure (HF) has shown efficacy both in acute and chronic settings. Recent percutaneous device innovations have pioneered a field known as interventional HF, providing clinicians with a variety of options for acute decompensated HF that are centered on nonsurgical mechanical circulatory support. Other structural-based therapies are aimed at the pathophysiology of chronic HF and target the underlying etiologies such as functional mitral regurgitation, ischemic cardiomyopathy, and increased neurohumoral activity. Remote hemodynamic monitoring devices have also been shown to be efficacious for the ambulatory management of HF. We review the current data on devices and investigational therapies for HF management whereby pharmacotherapy falls short.

Refractory angina (RA) is defined as chest pain caused by coronary ischemia in patients on maximal medical therapy and not amenable to revascularization despite advanced coronary artery disease (CAD). The long-term prognosis has improved with optimal medical therapy including risk factor modification. Still, patients are left with major impairment in quality of life and have high resource utilization with limited treatment options. We review the novel invasive and noninvasive therapies under investigation for RA.

Pulmonary arterial hypertension is a common and highly morbid medical problem resulting in elevated pulmonary arterial pressures and pulmonary vascular resistance. Medical therapies are costly, and not always well-tolerated. Surgical therapies such as pulmonary endarterectomy and lung transplantation are limited to a small subset of patients due to various patient, disease, or institutional factors. Over the past decade, there has been growing investigation into endovascular interventional therapies for patients with pulmonary hypertension such as balloon pulmonary angioplasty and pulmonary denervation. In this review, we describe the current status, future directions, and our recommendations on technical considerations with these therapies.

Pelvic venous disorders are inter-related pathologic conditions caused by reflux and obstruction in the pelvic veins. It can present a spectrum of clinical features based on the route of transmission of venous hypertension to either distal or caudal venous reservoirs. Imaging can help to visualize pelvic vascular and visceral structures to rule out other gynecologic, gastrointestinal, and urologic diseases. Endovascular treatment, owing to its low invasive nature and high success rate, has become the mainstay in the management of pelvic venous disorders. This article reviews the pathophysiology, clinical presentations, and diagnostic and therapeutic approaches to pelvic venous disorders.

> The severe acute respiratory syndrome coronavirus-2 (SARS-CoV-2) is a highly contagious pathogen resulting in the 2019 coronavirus disease (COVID-19) pandemic with direct impact on cardiac catheterization laboratory (CCL) operations. Initially, major challenges in limiting the spread of aerosolized pathogens existed until protocols were implemented to limit infectivity to staff and patients. COVID-19 increases the risk of myocardial infarctions and cardiogenic shock requiring acute management in the CCL. In this review, we specify best practices in the CCL for the management of infected patients in the preprocedure, intraprocedure, and postprocedure environments harmonizing available evidence, recommendations from international heart associations, and consensus opinion.

> Acute ischemic stroke (AIS) is one of the major causes of death worldwide and a leading cause of disability. Until recently treatment of AIS was supportive, and in a minority of patients intravenous thrombolysis was available but with marginal clinical benefit. With the advent of stent retrievers, distal aspiration catheters as well as improved patient selection neurologic outcomes have greatly improved. However, the care of patients with AIS is still challenging and requires the early recognition of stroke symptoms, extensive diagnostic testing, early intervention, and advanced nursing and critical care.

> Intracardiac and intravascular thrombi are associated with significant morbidity and mortality. Although surgery remains the gold standard treatment option, these patients often have multiple comorbidities that can make surgical options challenging. With advancements in catheter-based technologies, there are now percutaneous treatment options for these patients. The AngioVac is a percutaneous vacuum-assisted thrombectomy device FDA-approved for removal of intravascular debris that uses a venovenous extracorporeal membranous oxygenation circuit with a filter. Use of this device has now been reported in the removal of right atrial or iliocaval thrombi, debulking tricuspid vegetations, removal of vegetations from implantable cardiac devices, and pulmonary embolism.

SPECIAL TOPICS IN INTERVENTIONAL CARDIOLOGY

RELATED SERIES

Cardiology Clinics
Heart Failure Clinics
Cardiac Electrophysiology Clinics

THE CLINICS ARE NOW AVAILABLE ONLINE!

Access your subscription at:
www.theclinics.com

FOREWORD

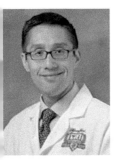

Marvin H. Eng, MD
Consulting Editor

We are pleased to introduce this latest issue of *Interventional Cardiology Clinics*, a compilation of topics germane to modern interventionalists but without an overarching theme sufficient for an entire issue. Therefore, we have compiled them as a "Special Topics" issue to address such orphan subjects. With the constant utilization of catheterization lab services and an increasingly broadening repertoire of interventional cardiologists, the cardiac catheterization lab is becoming the point of treatment for a myriad of unique clinical challenges.

Diversity is the theme, as this issue covers topics ranging from catheterization lab management during an infectious pandemic to the catheter-based management of heart failure. Technical subjects, such as paravalvular leak repair and use of electrosurgery in percutaneous procedures, are covered. More conceptual subjects, such as management of refractory angina and the role of pelvic venous disorders in heart failure, are explored in depth. New devices for vegetation and thrombus evacuation are covered as well as older procedures like alcohol septal ablation for hypertrophic obstructive cardiomyopathy. Given the occasional acute cerebrovascular event that occurs in the lab, we have invited experts to provide an update on acute neurointervention for ischemic stroke.

This issue provides comprehensive reviews for these diverse topics, and readers should find them enlightening. With a combination of established and new procedures, this issue should fill knowledge gaps of some of up-trending interventional dilemmas.

Marvin H. Eng, MD
Banner University Medical Center
1111 East, McDowell Road
Phoenix, AZ 85006, USA

E-mail address:
engm@email.arizona.edu

Intervent Cardiol Clin 11 (2022) xi
https://doi.org/10.1016/j.iccl.2022.04.001
2211-7458/22/© 2022 Published by Elsevier Inc.

Percutaneous Paravalvular Leak Repair

Marvin H. Eng, MD[a,b,*], Varun Tandon, MD[a], Adam B. Greenbaum, MD[c], Kenith Fang, MD[d]

KEYWORDS

- Percutaneous • Paravalvular leak • Aortic regurgitation • Mitral regurgitation

---

KEY POINTS

- Aortic paravalvular leaks (PVLs) can be grouped into transcatheter heart valve (THV) or surgical prosthesis lesions with the former having more options for treatment than the latter.
- Mitral PVLs are largely surgical with a small but growing population of THV procedure leaks.
- Advanced imaging is a vital component of defect localization and procedural guidance.
- Although not exhaustive, a suggested framework for trnascatheter PVL repair is defect localization, access planning, defect crossing, sheath delivery and occluder deployment. Detailed planning will facilitate the procedure, but operators must begin the case with a flexible mindset because many initial strategies may fail.

INTRODUCTION

Valve replacement is commonly performed either via surgery or using transcatheter technology. Although most valve replacements are efficacious, occasionally the implants are imperfect and paravalvular leaks (PVLs) manifest. PVL develop in 7-17% and 5-10% of surgical mitral and aortic valve replacements, respectively.[1,2] Contemporary data (2016–2019) from the Society of Thoracic Surgeon-American College of Cardiology transcatheter valve therapeutics registry reported a 1.6-2% rate of moderate-severe transcatheter aortic valve replacement (TAVR) PVL.[3] Operative mortality after TAVR ranges from 17.1-20% whereas reoperations for surgical PVL carry an 8.8-11.5% 30-day/in-hospital mortality.[4–8] Despite reoperation for surgical PVL, there is a 16-37% rate of recurrence of PVLs over time.[5–7] Owing to the hazards of surgical management of PVL, percutaneous repair has become a remedy.

PVL repairs are complex procedures that occur infrequently. Repairing PVL requires a thorough understanding of native and surgical anatomy, multimodality imaging, and catheter techniques. Owing to the complex nature of the procedures, there is a significant learning curve to the procedure, and it is usually reserved for experienced interventionalists. Increased experience reduced procedure time, contrast utilization, radiation exposure, length of stay, and major adverse cardiac events (MACE).[9] Retrospective comparison of transcatheter PVL closure with repeat surgery reveals an increased rate of major in-hospital morbidity for surgical cases (39.7%), but 30-day and 1-year mortalities were similar.[10] Similarly, another report showed higher technical success and in-hospital MACE for patients undergoing surgery when compared with patients receiving transcatheter therapies.[11,12] Again, mortality was similar for patients receiving transcatheter therapies and those undergoing surgery in this analysis.

---

[a] Division of Cardiology, Banner University Medical Center, 755 East McDowell Road, Phoenix, AZ 85006, USA; [b] Structural Heart Program, University of Arizona, Banner University Medical Center, 755 East McDowell Road, Phoenix, AZ 85006, USA; [c] Emory Structural Heart and Valve Center, 550 Peachtree Street, NE, Atlanta, GA 30308, USA; [d] Division of Cardiothoracic Surgery, Banner University Medical Center, 1111 East McDowell, Phoneix, AZ 85006, USA
* Corresponding author. Structural Heart Program, University of Arizona, Banner University Medical Center, 755 East McDowell Road, Phoenix, AZ 85006.
E-mail address: marvin.eng@bannerhealth.com

Intervent Cardiol Clin 11 (2022) 233–243
https://doi.org/10.1016/j.iccl.2022.03.004
2211-7458/22/© 2022 Published by Elsevier Inc.

Abbreviations

AoV	Aortic Valve
AR	Aortic Regurgitation
ARI	Aortic Regurgitation Index
CHAI	Composite Heart Rate Adjusted Hemodynamic-Echocardiographic Aortic Insufficiency Score
CT	Computed Tomography
F	French
ICE	Intracardiac Echocardiography
IAS	Intra-Atrial Septum
LAA	Left Atrial Appendage
LVOT	Left Ventricular Outflow Tract
MACE	Major Adverse Cardiac Events
PVL	Paravalvular Leak
PND	Paroxysmal Nocturnal Dyspnea
TIAR	Time-Integrated Aortic Regurgitation Index
THV	Transcatheter Heart Valve
TAVR	Transcatheter Aortic Valve Replacement
TEE	Transesophageal Echocardiography
TTE	Transthoracic Echocardiography
TMVR	Transcatheter Mitral Valve Replacement
ViV	Valve-in-Valve
ViR	Valve-in-Ring
VSD	Ventricular Septal Defect

Contemporary outcomes with PVL closure differ depending on leak location, results achieved after closure, and urgency of treatment. Aortic PVL is associated with a 90-93.1% rate of success, and if mild or less leaking is achieved, the event-free survival at 2 years is 98%.[12,13] Mitral PVL is associated with a lower success rate (70.1–86%).[11,13] Predictors of MACE and death with PVL repair includes age, urgency of presentation, renal function, New York Heart Association class, and leak severity. The only independent predictor of death is leak severity at follow-up.[13] Of note mitral PVL was associated with a higher rate of MACE (1.83 hazard ratio [1.15–2.91]; $P = .01$). New hemolysis post-PVL closure has only been documented to be 1.6% in 1 multicenter registry and remains a minor concern when performing repairs.[13] There are a myriad of reasons for transcatheter PVL failure, some that are specific to surgical valves (Box 1) but others that are universal to transcatheter heart valves (THVs) and surgical prosthetics.[9]

Clinical evaluation for suspected PVL: Complete past medical history including detailed surgical or transcatheter implantation history should be obtained. Patients with a history of endocarditis are particularly prone to developing PVL postoperatively.[6] A history of heart failure symptoms, primarily dyspnea, paroxysmal nocturnal dyspnea (PND), or lower extremity edema should trigger concern for a PVL. The natural history of valves shows that PVLs can appear over time and there need not be an early

Box 1
Reasons for procedural failure for paravalvular leak closure

Reasons for procedural failure

Prosthetic leaflet impingement

Residual regurgitation despite device deployment

Device embolization

Inability to cross with guidewire

Inability to cross with delivery sheath

Coronary dissection

Table 1
Options for treating aortic paravalvular leak based on prosthesis type

	Surgical	Transcatheter
Redo surgery	X	X
Balloon dilation		X
Valve-in-valve	X	X
Transcatheter repair	X	X

surgical failure for PVLs to appear.[2] The appearance of dark or brown urine should prompt concerns over hemolysis. Physical examination detection of murmurs or signs of congestions such as rales, jugular venous distention, or lower extremity edema should prompt further investigation. Standard evaluation for heart failure should occur with chest radiography and laboratory studies, but a survey for possible endocarditis should be performed in new bioprosthetic valve regurgitation. If examining for hemolysis, then laboratory studies should include serum hemoglobin, plasma-free hemoglobin, lactate dehydrogenase, bilirubin, haptoglobulin, peripheral smear, and reticulocyte count.

To simplify the approach, PVL repair should be partitioned according to location. While PVL can develop position with a prosthesis, the focus of this review is the approach to transcatheter aortic and mitral PVL closure.

Aortic Paravalvular Leak
Assessment and approach
Aortic PVL cases should first be grouped into either TAVR or surgical PVL, because there are more options for treating the former. If not a surgical candidate, TAVR PVL can be treated with postdilation of the THV, valve-in-valve (ViV) TAVR, or transcatheter PVL repair (Table 1). Balloon postdilation of THV was able to reduce moderate to severe PVL by 15-fold, but it did not reduce PVL to the same rates as patients who did not require postdilation.[14] Surgical PVL can only be treated with repeat surgery, transcatheter PVL repair, and in some instances, ViV-TAVR with bioprosthetic fracture.[15] As the techniques of postdilation and ViV TAVR are relatively straightforward, this review focuses on PVL repair.

As mentioned previously, transcatheter PVL repair is a procedure that involves a significant learning curve and unique challenges that can occur from case to case. Although this review is not an exhaustive exploration of all the possible PVL repair techniques, it highlights the salient decisions required during cases and is hoped to provide a framework for approaching PVL repair cases.

Noninvasive imaging
This imaging is usually performed with both transthoracic echocardiography (TTE) and transesophageal echocardiography (TEE). Recently the American Society of Echocardiography has revised its grading scheme and includes percentage circumference of the prosthesis in characterization of PVL severity.[16] The entirety of PVL gradient by echocardiography extends beyond the scope of this review. Computed tomographic (CT) scan can assist with anatomically localizing the defect and understanding character of the tract because some PVLs may involve aneurysms of the aortic root.

The most important step is localization of the defect. Conceptualization of the PVL locations should revolve around the aortic prosthesis and subdividing the perimeter into the native coronary cusp anatomy (Fig. 1). The non, left, and right coronary cusps help orient clinicians to the prosthesis and defect location. Localizing the defect according to a cusp helps to locate the defect to a more anterior/posterior or lateral location and helps operators find an appropriate viewing projection to facilitate defect crossing. Therefore by orienting lesions according to coronary cusps, catheter selection should be based on shapes that routinely aim toward the specific coronary cusp (eg, Extra-Backup Guide for the left coronary cusp).

Invasive Evaluation
Hemodynamic assessment using the pulse pressure index may be of assistance, and there have been several iterations to corroborate significance of hemodynamic disturbances to mortality (Table 2).[17–20] In addition, the presence of pulmonary hypertension may corroborate the

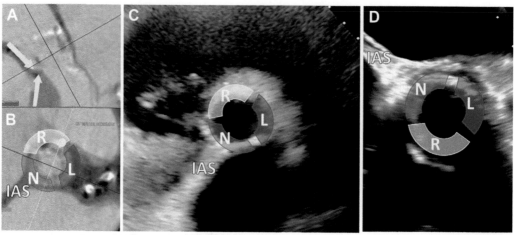

Fig. 1. Conceptualized aortic anatomy to facilitate paravalvular leak closure. (*A*) CT of the aortic bioprosthesis. A breach in the region by the right coronary cusp (*arrows*) is noted and is the source of this surgical paravalvular leak. (*B*) En face anatomy of the aortic valve prosthesis with the right, left, and noncoronary cusps of the aortic valve by CT. (*C*) TTE short-axis view of the aortic prosthesis mirrors the orientation of the CT scan. (*D*) TEE of the aortic prosthesis again illustrating right, left, and noncoronary cusp orientation, but the typical convention is for anterior to be closer to the bottom of the image because the probe is imaging from the esophagus, a structure posterior to the heart. In general, paravalvular leaks should be localized accordingly to cross the defect with more precision. IAS, intra-atrial septum; L, left coronary cusp; N, noncoronary cusp; R, right coronary cusp.

severity of the aortic regurgitation. Aortography may be used to confirm regurgitation severity based on the Sellers criteria.

Access

Size of the access should be proportionate to the size of the defect. If the defect is anticipated to require more than 1 closure device, then it may be preferable to use a larger sheath so long as the vessel can accommodate its size. Most frequently a femoral approach is used, and if several devices are anticipated, then use of a larger bore Gore DrySeal (12F–16F) (Gore Medical, Flagstaff, AZ, USA) should be considered to accommodate multiple catheters. In such cases then a vascular closure plan should be in place to either use Perclose ProGlide (Abbott Vascular, Santa Clara, AZ, USA) or MANTA (Teleflex Medicine, Wayne, PA, USA).

Baseline Assessment

Characterization of the leak and hemodynamic status should be performed. Frequently, aortography with a 20- to 30-mL injection should suffice.

Table 2
Hemodynamic indexes used to assess paravalvular leak severity

Author	Index	Formula	Cutoff for Significance
Sinning et al[17]	AR index	([DBP-LVEDP]÷SBP) × 100	AR index <25 predicted higher mortality
Sinning et al[18]	ARI ratio	Ratio of postprocedural to preprocedural AR index	ARI ratio <0.60 improved 1-y mortality prediction of post-TAVR AR index <25
Jilaihawi et al[19]	CHAI score	([DBP-LVEDP] ÷HR) × 80	<25 (denoted ≥ moderate PVR), predicted higher mortality
Bugan et al[20]	TIAR index	(LV-Ao diastolic pressure time integral)/(LV systolic pressure time integral) × 100	TIAR index < 80 was associated with a sensitivity of 86% and a specificity of 83% for ≥ mild AR

AR, aortic regurgitation; ARI, aortic regurgitation index; CHAI, Composite heart rate adjusted hemodynamic-echocardiographic aortic insufficiency score; TIAR, time-integrated aortic regurgitation index

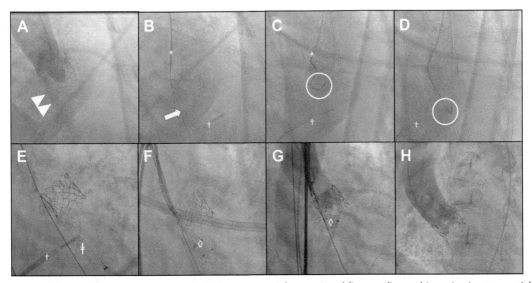

Fig. 2. Aortic PVL closure. (A) Aortography in an extreme right anterior oblique radiographic projection tangential to the leak and demonstrates the jet is posterior (*arrowheads*). (B) A 7F Extra-Backup (EBU) guide and 4F Berenstein catheter in a mother/daughter configuration (*asterisk*) directing a straight stiff glidewire through the defect (*arrow*). An intracardiac echo (ICE) catheter is present. (C, D) The glidewire is snared (*circle*) to provide countertraction and facilitate crossing of the Berenstein catheter (*asterisk*). (E) Exchange was made for a 0.035-in Super Stiff Amplatz wire and facilitate crossing of 6F shuttle sheaths (*double dagger*). (F, G) Two sheaths are delivered and two 4-mm ventricular septal defect (VSD) occluders are deployed in the PVL (*diamond*). (H) Final aortography demonstrates obliteration of the PVL and resolution of aortic regurgitation. Dagger, intra-cardiac echocardiography probe

Based on TTE/TEE findings and possibly CT projection modeling, an angiographic view can be estimated that provides a tangential perspective of the leak to facilitate crossing. If renal insufficiency does not enable the use of contrast, then the operator will need to exclusively rely on echocardiography Most cases use TEE, but some have used intracardiac echocardiography (ICE) to assess aortic insufficiency and guide the procedure.[21] For cases with a mechanical prosthesis, a cineangiographic run of the baseline functioning mechanical leaflets should be performed.

Hemodynamic assessment of the simultaneous left ventricular and aortic pressures along with right heart catheterization is preferred. Baseline aortic and left ventricular pressures should be measured as there are rare instances where the disk of a closure device can increase left ventricular outflow tract (LVOT) gradients.

Defect crossing
Defect crossing is sometimes extremely challenging and often the crux of a successful procedure (Figs. 2 and 3). The use of mother-daughter catheter systems to direct a long (400 cm) straight stiff glidewire (Terumo, Ann Arbor, MI, USA) is the most direct means of traversing paravalvular defects. The mother catheter is usually a 7F coronary guide catheter.

The daughter catheter is usually a 4F to 5F long catheter (130–150 cm) and preferably hydrophilic coated. A long glidewire (400 cm) is preferred in the event an externalized rail is used to facilitate catheter delivery. Once the wire is across the defect, a tangential fluoroscopic viewing angle should be used to confirm crossing external to prosthetic valve.

Sheath/catheter delivery
Once the wire has traversed the defect, telescope the daughter catheter across. If there is difficulty in the daughter catheter traversal, then exchanging for a lower profile straight catheter (ie, Quick-Cross 0.035" [Spectranetics, Colorado Springs, CO, USA]) or snaring and externalizing the crossing wire to provide countertraction should be considered. The countertraction may come from the left ventricle via the aortic valve, transseptally or in rare cases, transapically. (see Figs. 2 and 3).

After daughter catheter traversal, the goal is to deliver a sheath for occluder placement (see Figs. 2 and 3). Sheaths are preferable to guide catheters because they can accommodate larger devices. At this point, the operator can choose to exchange for a stiff wire to facilitate death delivery. Otherwise, if using a rail, sheath can be delivered over the externalized wire and then

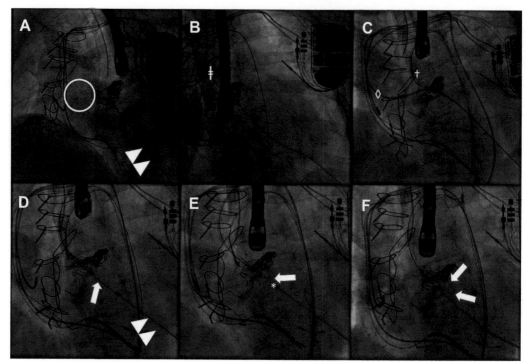

Fig. 3. Aortic PVL closure with the use of an apical rail. (*A*) A 6F sheath 23 cm has been placed percutaneously (*arrowheads*). A 6F JR4 guide has directed a 0.035-in stiff-angled glidewire (*circle*) across an aortic PVL in an antegrade fashion. Note that this PVL and the associated aortic pseudoaneurysm had previously been treated with an Amplatzer Vascular Plug (AVP) II and coils. (*B*) The 0.035-in wire was snared and externalized, creating a rail (*double dagger*) to facilitate sheath delivery. (*C*) The preexisting AVP II is snared (*dagger*) and retracted to enable sheath delivery. A 7F shuttle sheath is tracked over the glidewire rail (*diamond*); note that resistance to sheath traversal has resulted in bowing of the sheath toward the greater curvature of the aorta. (*D*) With the glidewire still present within the shuttle sheath, a 4-mm VSD occlude is deployed (*arrow*) and the apical sheath (*arrowheads*) remains. (*E*) The previously deployed VSD plug remains attached to the deployment cable (*arrow*), and a new VSD plug is being deployed (*asterisk*) through the shuttle sheath over the preexisting apical rail. (*F*) Both VSD plugs are present and deployed (*arrows*), and the operators prepare to dismantle the apical rail, remove the sheath, and hemostatically plug the apical access (not shown).

used to deliver as many devices as required (see Fig. 3). Alternatively, the sheath can deliver several stiff wires for several sheaths simultaneously and evenly space occluder device delivery (see Fig. 2).

Closure device selection

Closure devices should be selected according to the size of the defect (Table 3). Typically, the authors advise sizing the devices to be at least 1.5× the diameter of the defect. Some defects are crescentic in nature and require several devices. Occluders are most frequently made of Nitinol and have differing shapes, delivery sheath sizes, and weaves. Some occluder devices have cloth to assist in obliterating blood flow. Thus far there are no prospective or comparative data to confirm superior efficacy of one device over another.

Once the closure devices are in place and there is no longer any need for additional delivery sheath traversal, the rail can be removed. All the occluder device cables should remain connected until there is no longer a need to cross the defect with any catheters or sheaths.

Outcome assessment

Once the maximal number of devices have delivered, repeat assessment of the leak with echocardiography/angiography and hemodynamics is reocmmended (see Fig. 2). Mechanical valves require repeat functional assessment of the leaflets by echocardiography or fluoroscopy. When coronary vessels are in close proximity, patency should be reconfirmed. Once aortic insufficiency is sufficiently treated, all occluder devices can be released from their respective cables.

Postprocedure management should include serial testing for hemolysis including haptoglobulin, lactate dehydrogenase, plasma hemoglobin, and peripheral smear. Urine color and

Table 3
Commonly used occluder devices for paravalvular leak repair

Device	Range of Lobe Size (mm)	Disk Extend Lobe by (mm)	Sheath (F)	Considerations
Amplatzer Duct Occluder	5–12	4–6	5–7	Device length is only 5–8 mm
Amplatzer Duct Occluder II	3–6	6	4–5	3-lobed device, 2 outer disks and 1 inner lobe
Occlutech PDA Occluder	3.5–14	5.5–10	6–8	Lobe is conical with the proximal end 1.5–4 mm larger; OUS only
Amplatzer Muscular VSD Occluder	4–18	5–8	5–9	Waist length 7 mm, very stiff device
Amplatzer Septal Occluder	4–38	12–16	6–12	Left atrial disc > right atrial disc diameter
Amplatzer Vascular Plug II	3–22	0	4–7	Most frequently used device for large defects
Amplatzer Vascular Plug III	4 ×2–14 ×5	2	4–7	Difficult to orient when collapsed
Amplatzer Vascular Plug IV	4–8	N/A	4F diagnostic catheter	Suited for small PVL

OUS, Outside of the United States; N/A, not available.

consistency should be noted, and if there is hemolysis, then the patient should be adequately hydrated to prevent pigment nephropathy.

Troubleshooting

For very difficult crossing, sometimes 0.014-in wires have been used to cross defects and serial exchanges used to deliver sheaths. In addition, at times, some have used antegrade crossing from a transseptal or apical access to cross a defect. Some defects that are difficult to traverse with sheaths have required balloon assist tracking to cross. It should be noted that extreme care should be used for patients with paravalvular TAVR leaks because forceful sheath delivery can dislodge a THV possibly resulting in dire consequences.

Mitral Paravalvular Leaks

At present, most mitral PVLs are surgical in nature; however, transcatheter mitral valve replacement (TMVR) PVLs are beginning to grow as a cohort. Transcatheter mitral valve-in-ring (ViR) and transcatheter mitral valve in mitral annular calcification (ViMAC) procedures are currently sources of paravalvular leaks. Although there are no US Food and Drug Administration-approved devices for native TMVR, it is anticipated that a low rate of PVL will likely surface once the technology is disseminated.

As previously mentioned, PVL repair is complex and given the documented lower success rates of mitral PVL closure, planning is even more vital to success.[11] Again, perhaps the most important facet of achieving success is defect localization because there are sometimes multiple defects around a single prosthesis (Fig. 4). For mitral anatomic localization, use of 3D-TEE is incredibly helpful, nearly indispensable. In fact, the efficiencies gained over the evolution of PVL repair have been attributed to implementation of 3D-TEE.[9] If using 3D TEE, the aorta should be conveniently oriented such that it approximates 12-o'clock position, the left atrial appendage 9-o'clock position, and the atrial septum 3-o'clock position (see Fig. 4). Once localized, further plans for transseptal access, steerable guide, daughter catheter selection, and whether to use a rail should be decided. Of note, CT has comparable sensitivity and specificity for identifying PVL as 3D-TEE and both modalities can be helpful for planning.[22]

Access

Most mitral PVL repairs are performed via transseptal access; however, a small proportion has been done via a limited thoracotomy and transapical access.[23,24] A large-bore sheath should be used, typically from the right femoral vein.

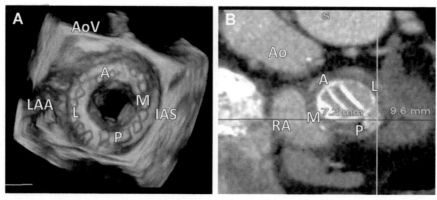

Fig. 4. Mitral valve anatomy orientation to facilitate mitral PVL closure. (A) Left atrial view of the mitral valve typical for transcatheter interventions orienting the aortic valve at the top of the screen, the left atrial appendage (LAA) to the left, and intra-atrial septum (IAS) to the right. (B) CT scan of a mechanical mitral valve with a posterior PVL. Note the orientation of the mitral annulus and the posterior PVL dimensions of 7.2 × 9.6 mm. A, anterior; AoV, aortic valve; L, lateral; M, medial; P, posterior; RA, right atrium.

Again, a Gore DrySeal can facilitate the use of several catheters or guides, and the size depends on the size of the leak. As venous access is usually much more forgiving, use of a larger sheath has less risk for vascular complications than with arterial access.

Baseline assessment

Just as in aortic PVLs, a baseline hemodynamic and leak severity assessment should be completed. Right heart catheterization, left atrial pressure and a direct transmitral gradient should be measured. For anterior leaks, baseline left

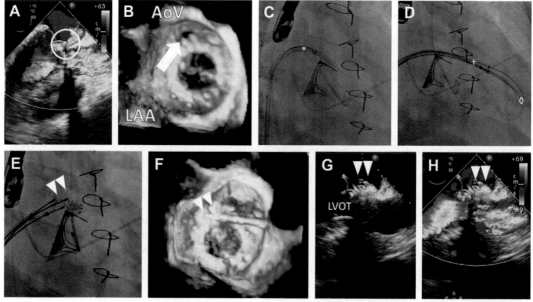

Fig. 5. Mitral PVL closure. (A) TEE with color Doppler demonstrating an anterior mitral PVL (circle) at the aorto-mitral curtain. (B) 3D-TEE confirming an anterior PVL (arrow). Note its relationship to the aortic valve (AoV). (C) A medium curl Agilis catheter (Abbott Vascular, Santa Cruz, CA, USA) and 5F Berenstein catheter in a mother/daughter (asterisk) configuration directs a straight stiff glidewire across the defect. (D) Traversal of the defect with several shuttle sheaths (dagger) via several Super-Stiff Amplatz wires (diamond). (E) Two 4-mm VSD and 6-mm Amplatzer Duct Occluder (ADO) II occluders (arrowheads) are deployed in the PVL tract. (F) 3D-TEE visualization of the occluder devices (arrowheads) and the deployment cables. (G, H) 2D-TEE confirmation of the occluder devices (arrowheads) not encroaching upon the left ventricular outflow tract (LVOT). Doppler interrogation (H) confirms obliteration of the PVL with cessation of color flow.

ventricle-aortic pressure gradient should be measured because plugs that encroach upon the LVOT could elevate the gradient. Leak severity can be documented by TEE, or if renal function is adequate, ventriculography can be performed. Again, if a mechanical prosthesis is present, baseline functioning of the leaflets should be documented.

Adjunctive imaging

At present, TEE is most frequently used for procedural guidance with some exceptions for operators who may use ICE. 3D imaging is nearly indispensable for image guidance improves efficiency significantly. Again, orienting the mitral prosthesis so that the aorta approximates 12-o'clock position facilitates navigation and PVL crossing in the left atrium. The process of navigation requires the imaging physician and proceduralist to synchronize with respect to anatomic orientation and catheter manipulation to have clear communication during the case; this needs to be established early in the case. Some centers use fluoroscopy/echocardiographic fusion technology to facilitate closure.[25] Also, 4D ICE may eventually supplant 3D-TEE for image guidance and obviate general anesthesia, minimizing resource utilization for these complex procedures.

Crossing

Recommended strategy for the antegrade crossing of a mitral PVL involves using a deflectable sheath, a hydrophilic catheter, and a hydrophilic wire (Fig. 5). An example of such a system would be an Agilis medium curl sheath, Berenstein catheter, and a straight stiff glidewire, but several permutations of catheters and wire can be chosen. The essential concept is to create a serial, telescoping system supportive enough to deliver a sheath across the PVL (see Fig. 5). The leaks can be crossed in a retrograde fashion as well, but this is less commonly performed.

Once across, the operators will need to decide if countertraction will be necessary (see Fig. 5). For difficult-to-traverse paravalvular tracts, sometimes additional support is needed for sheath delivery. In these cases, the additional support can be gained by using either telescoping through a large 12F to 14F deflectable sheath (eg, FlexCath [Medtronic, St Paul, MN, USA]) or providing countertraction from the distal side of the wire from the ventricular side. The source of the countertraction most frequently comes from the aorta, but there are rare instances when transapical access provides the best source of countertraction (see Fig. 3).

Once across, the operator will again need to decide how many devices will be necessary and decide on either delivering multiple sheaths across or serially deploying devices over a stiff wire until the leak is sufficiently treated (see Figs. 3 and 5).

Outcome assessment

After satisfactory treatment of the defect, echocardiographic or angiographic quantification of the regurgitation should be performed (see Fig. 5). Pulmonary and left atrial pressure hemodynamic assessment should be repeated. If treating defects near the aortic valve or LVOT, repeat assessment should be performed including LVOT gradient and aortic valve functioning because these could be compromised from occluder disk placement. Mechanical prosthesis leaflet functioning should be reevaluated, and if all are satisfactory, then the devices can be released from the delivery cables.

Troubleshooting

Similar to aortic PVL challenges, use of 0.014-in wires or crossing retrograde from the ventricle can sometimes be helpful. Difficult delivery sheath traversal may prompt balloon-assisted tracking to facilitate crossing at the expense of possibly making the leak worse. Treatment of TMVR ViR PVL will be more complex because the point of breach is a dehisced ring. In addition, crossing such a leak is complicated because wires may traverse through an open cell of the THV and if unrecognized, occlude devices that may be deployed within the cage of the THV. Of note, freshly implanted occluder devices can be retrieved with snares and removed. At times when revising a failed PVL closure, it is usually better to remove the ineffective occluders and start over because device choice or suboptimal deployment may have been part of the failure.

SUMMARY

Transcatheter PVL repair is complex and requires an in-depth understanding of surgical and transcatheter therapies, multimodality imaging, and transcatheter techniques for crossing and delivering devices. Of transcatheter therapies, it represents one of the most advanced procedures to attempt and is usually reserved for highly experienced teams of imagers and operators. Most importantly, proceduralists must remain flexible when attempting these procedures and allow for secondary plans should the initial strategy be thwarted. Future advances in transcatheter PVL repair include more experience with 4D ICE, more efficacious occluder devices, and nuanced techniques for treatment of TMVR PVL. Although it would be optimistic to believe that upcoming valve therapies will make such repairs obsolete, everything will have a certain degree of failure and PVL repair is likely to remain one of the most advanced procedures in a team's repertoire.

CLINICS CARE POINTS

- Thorough assessment of PVL anatomy needs to be performed with a combination of echocardiography and frequently with CT to localize the leak.
- Transcatheter PVL repair requires detailed planning in a structured manner that should include defect localization, access, defect crossing, sheath delivery, and occluder deployment

DISCLOSURE

M.H. Eng is a clinical proctor for Edwards Lifesciences and Medtronic. A.B. Greenbaum is a proctor for Edwards Lifesciences, and Medtronic. He is a consultant with equity in Transmural Systems. His employer has research contracts for investigation of aortic and mitral devices from Edwards Lifesciences, Abbott Vascular, Medtronic, and Boston Scientific. K. Fang is a consultant to Abbott Vascular and Atricure.

REFERENCES

1. Hammermeister K, Gulshan KS, Henderson WG, et al. Outcomes 15 years after valve replacement with a mechanical versus a bioprosthetic vavle: final report of the veterans affairs randomized trial. J Am Coll Cardiol 2000;36:1152–8.
2. Ionescu A, Fraser AG, Butchart EG. Prevalence and clinical significance of incidental paraprosthetic valvar regurgitation: a prospective study using transoesophageal echocardiography. Heart 2003;89:1316–21.
3. Carroll JD, Mack MJ, Vemulapalli S, et al. STS-ACC TVT Registry of Transcatheter Aortic Valve Replacement. J Am Coll Cardiol 2020;76:2492–516.
4. Jawitz OK, Gulack BC, Grau-Sepulveda MV, et al. Reoperation after transcatheter aortic valve replacement: an analysis of the society of thoracic surgeons database. JACC Cardiovasc Interv 2020;13:1515–25.
5. Choi JW, Hwang HY, Kim KH, et al. Long-term results of surgical correction for mitral paravalvular leak: repair versus re-replacement. J Heart Valve Dis 2013;22:682–7.
6. Taramasso M, Maisano F, Denti P, et al. Surgical treatment of paravalvular leak: Long-term results in a single-center experience (up to 14 years). J Thorac Cardiovasc Surg 2015;149:1270–5.
7. Akins CW, Bitondo JM, Hilgenberg AD, et al. Early and late results of the surgical correction of cardiac prosthetic paravalvular leaks. J Heart Valve Dis 2005;14:792–9 [discussion: 799-800].
8. Brescia AA, Deeb GM, Sang SLW, et al. Surgical explantation of transcatheter aortic valve bioprostheses: a Statewide Experience. Circ Cardiovasc Interv 2021;14:e009927.
9. Sorajja P, Cabalka AK, Hagler DJ, et al. The learning curve in percutaneous repair of paravalvular prosthetic regurgitation: an analysis of 200 cases. JACC Cardiovasc Interv 2014;7:521–9.
10. Wells JAt, Condado JF, Kamioka N, et al. Outcomes after paravalvular leak closure: transcatheter versus surgical approaches. JACC Cardiovasc Interv 2017;10:500–7.
11. Alkhouli M, Rihal CS, Zack CJ, et al. Transcatheter and surgical management of mitral paravalvular leak: long-term outcomes. JACC Cardiovasc Interv 2017;10:1946–56.
12. Alkhouli M, Sarraf M, Maor E, et al. Techniques and outcomes of percutaneous aortic paravalvular leak closure. JACC Cardiovasc Interv 2016;9:2416–26.
13. Calvert PA, Northridge DB, Malik IS, et al. Percutaneous device closure of paravalvular leak. Circulation 2016;134:934–44.
14. Wang N, Lal S. Post-dilation in transcatheter aortic valve replacement: a systematic review and meta-analysis. J Interv Cardiol 2017;30:204–11.
15. Loyalka P, Montgomery KB, Nguyen TC, et al. Valve-in-valve transcatheter aortic valve implantation: a novel approach to treat paravalvular leak. Ann Thorac Surg 2017;104:e325–7.
16. Zoghbi WA, Asch FM, Bruce C, et al. Guidelines for the Evaluation of Valvular Regurgitation After Percutaneous Valve Repair or Replacement: A Report from the American Society of Echocardiography Developed in Collaboration with the Society for Cardiovascular Angiography and Interventions, Japanese Society of Echocardiography, and Society for Cardiovascular Magnetic Resonance. J Am Soc Echocardiogr 2019;32:431–75.
17. Sinning JM, Hammerstingl C, Vasa-Nicotera M, et al. Aortic regurgitation index defines severity of peri-prosthetic regurgitation and predicts outcome in patients after transcatheter aortic valve implantation. J Am Coll Cardiol 2012;59:1134–41.
18. Sinning JM, Stundl A, Pingel S, et al. Pre-procedural hemodynamic status improves the discriminatory value of the aortic regurgitation index in patients undergoing

transcatheter aortic valve replacement. JACC Cardiovasc Interv 2016;9:700–11.

19. Jilaihawi H, Chakravarty T, Shiota T, et al. Heart-rate adjustment of transcatheter haemodynamics improves the prognostic evaluation of paravalvular regurgitation after transcatheter aortic valve implantation. EuroIntervention 2015;11:456–64.

20. Bugan B, Kapadia S, Svensson L, et al. Novel hemodynamic index for assessment of aortic regurgitation after transcatheter aortic valve replacement. Catheter Cardiovasc Interv 2015;86:E174–9.

21. Ruparelia N, Cao J, Newton JD, et al. Paravalvular leak closure under intracardiac echocardiographic guidance. Catheter Cardiovasc Interv 2018;91:958–65.

22. Suh YJ, Hong GR, Han K, et al. Assessment of mitral paravalvular leakage after mitral valve replacement using cardiac computed tomography: comparison with surgical findings. Circ Cardiovasc Imaging 2016;9.

23. Taramasso M, Maisano F, Latib A, et al. Conventional surgery and transcatheter closure via surgical transapical approach for paravalvular leak repair in high-risk patients: results from a single-centre experience. Eur Heart J Cardiovasc Imaging 2014; 15:1161–7.

24. Eng MH, Kherallah RY, Guerrero M, et al. Complete percutaneous apical access and closure: Short and intermediate term outcomes. Catheter Cardiovasc Interv 2020;96:481–7.

25. Jone PN, Haak A, Ross M, et al. Congenital and Structural Heart Disease Interventions Using Echocardiography-Fluoroscopy Fusion Imaging. J Am Soc Echocardiogr 2019;32:1495–504.

26. Nietlispach F, Maisano F, Sorajja P, et al. Percutaneous paravalvular leak closure: chasing the chameleon. Eur Heart J 2016;37:3495–502.

Alcohol Septal Ablation for Obstructive Hypertrophic Cardiomyopathy

Paul Sorajja, MD[a,b,c],*, Robert Fraser, MD[a,c], Robert Steffen, MD[a,c], Kevin M. Harris, MD[a,c]

KEYWORDS

- Hypertrophic obstructive cardiomyopathy • Alcohol septal ablation • Myomectomy
- Percutaneous

KEY POINTS

- For alcohol septal ablation to be effective, left ventricular outflow obstruction must be from systolic thickening of the ventricular septum and associated with systolic anterior mitral leaflet motion.
- National guidelines for alcohol septal ablation have emphasized patients who are high risk or inoperable for surgery and the prerequisite for institutional and operator experience.
- The most common complication of alcohol septal ablation is heart block. Rate of pacemaker dependency postablation is 10% for patients with a normal ECG and up to 50% with baseline QRS widening or severe left axis deviation.

INTRODUCTION

Since the first reports of alcohol septal ablation (ASA) for hypertrophic cardiomyopathy (HCM) in 1995, the procedure has become established for selected patients with drug-refractory symptoms due to dynamic left ventricular outflow tract (LVOT) obstruction.[1] The premise of ASA is catheter-based injection of alcohol into one or more septal perforator arteries and the creation of a controlled myocardial infarction of the ventricular septum that relieves dynamic LVOT obstruction. Procedural success depends highly on appropriate patient selection and operator experience, ideally in the setting of a comprehensive center dedicated to the longitudinal care of patients with HCM.

DYNAMIC LEFT VENTRICULAR OUTFLOW TRACT OBSTRUCTION

Dynamic LVOT obstruction occurs in ~75% of patients with HCM.[1] Two main mechanisms precipitate the development of obstruction in these patients: (1) septal hypertrophy with outflow tract narrowing leads to Venturi forces that accelerate during ventricular emptying and draw the mitral valvular apparatus anteriorly and (2) anterior papillary muscle displacement that subjects the mitral leaflets to intraventricular currents during systole that drag the apparatus anteriorly. The loss of mitral leaflet coaptation also leads to valvular regurgitation, which is dynamic and temporally related to onset of LVOT obstruction. Both the LVOT and associated mitral regurgitation are dynamic,

---

[a] Center for Valve and Structural Heart Disease, Minneapolis Heart Institute at Abbott Northwestern Hospital, 920 East, 28th Street, Minneapolis, MN 55417, USA; [b] Valve Science Center, Minneapolis Heart Institute Foundation, Abbott Northwestern Hospital, 800 East 28th Street, Minneapolis, MN 55401, USA; [c] Hypertrophic Cardiomyopathy Center, Minneapolis Heart Institute Foundation, 920 East, 28th Street, Minneapolis, MN 55417, USA
* Corresponding author.
E-mail addresses: paul.sorajja@allina.com; psorajja@gmail.com

and depend on the preload, afterload, and contractile state of the left ventricle. The obstruction may be present in the resting state, present only during provocation, or absent.

PATIENT SELECTION

The therapeutic goal of ASA is symptom relief by reducing systolic thickening of the ventricular septum that is responsible for dynamic LVOT obstruction and associated mitral regurgitation. Candidate patients are those with (1) severe, drug-refractory cardiovascular symptoms, including dyspnea, angina class, or disabling presyncope or syncope; (2) dynamic LVOT obstruction due to systolic anterior motion of the mitral valve (gradient ≥30 mm Hg at rest or ≥50 mm Hg with provocation); (3) ventricular septal thickness greater than or equal to 15 mm; (4) suitable coronary anatomy; (5) no significant intrinsic mitral valve disease; and (5) absence of need for concomitant cardiac surgical procedure (eg, valve replacement, bypass grafting). In general, patients with severe myocardial hypertrophy (eg, septal thickness >25 mm) should not be treated with ASA due to the large doses of alcohol required.

For informed consent, a shared decision-making process should be used with a comprehensive discussion of all therapeutic options, including ASA, medical therapy, and surgical myectomy. In this discussion, it is important to note the standard of surgical myectomy, which is successful in greater than 90% and associated with an operative mortality of less than 1%, when performed on appropriate surgical patients in experienced centers.[2] Risks of ASA, including pacemaker dependency (see later discussion) and other catheter-based complications, should be discussed in detail.

Comprehensive imaging with 2D and Doppler echocardiography is essential for appropriate selection. In order for ASA to be effective, LVOT obstruction should be dynamic, arising from systolic thickening of the ventricular septum, and accompanied by systolic anterior motion of the mitral valve at rest or with provocation. The jet of mitral regurgitation associated with dynamic LVOT obstruction is posterior; the presence of central or anterior mitral regurgitation should raise the suspicion of intrinsic valve disease (eg, flail segment or myxomatous degeneration) (Fig. 1). In patients with posterior mitral regurgitation, excessive leaflet tethering from secondary causes (eg, ischemic cardiomyopathy) should be excluded. For determining the LVOT gradient, particular care should be undertaken to distinguish the Doppler signal of obstruction from

that of mitral regurgitation. For cases in which the severity of the LVOT gradient cannot be determined noninvasively, cardiac catheterization should be performed. During coronary angiography, suitability of coronary anatomy should be determined from studies of both the left and the right coronary artery, from which proximal septal perforators can arise.

For patient selection for ASA, national guidelines have emphasized the importance of operator and institutional expertise, preference for patients who are either at high risk or inoperable for surgery, and avoidance in patients who either have massive hypertrophy or who are relatively young (Box 1).[3] In these guidelines, an experienced operator is defined as a person with a cumulative case volume of 20 procedures or more or one who is working in a dedicated HCM program with a cumulative experience of 50 procedures or more. The operator must have comprehensive skills in interpretation of echocardiographic findings of HCM for both planning and execution of the procedure, as well as the postoperative care.

PROCEDURAL TECHNIQUES

ASA may be performed under general anesthesia or conscious sedation. With conscious sedation and use of transthoracic echocardiography for imaging, patients may be able to perform the Valsalva maneuver for assessing the dynamic nature of the LVOT obstruction, and patient recovery is expedited. For general anesthesia, transesophageal echocardiography facilitates excellent visualization of the basal ventricular septum, which can be obscured during contrast echocardiography using transthoracic imaging. General anesthesia also facilitates patient analgesia for discomfort related to the iatrogenic myocardial infarction, as well as transesophageal imaging for transseptal puncture and hemodynamic catheterization.

Temporary Pacemaker Placement

Owing to the potential for complete heart block, all patients without prior permanent pacemaker implantation should undergo temporary pacemaker placement, typically via internal jugular venous access to enable both backup pacing and ambulation in the postoperative period. Occurrence of permanent pacemaker dependency from ASA varies according to the baseline conduction abnormalities. The area of iatrogenic infarction usually courses inferiorly from the junction of the anterior and inferior septum toward the right ventricular side of the ventricular septum.[4] This area frequently contains the right

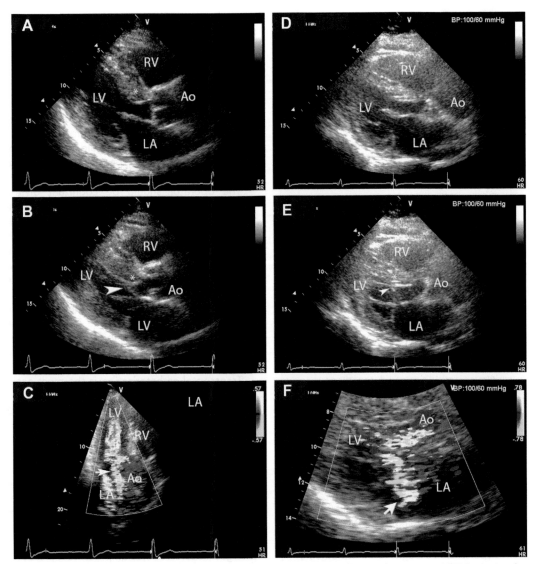

Fig. 1. Dynamic LVOT obstruction and associated mitral regurgitation in HCM. (*Left*) Parasternal long-axis view from transthoracic echocardiography showing hypertrophy (*top, arrow*) and dynamic LVOT obstruction with systolic anterior motion of the mitral valve (*middle, arrowhead*) and mitral regurgitation. However, the direction of the mitral jet is anterior, demonstrating the presence of intrinsic mitral disease that would not benefit from alcohol septal ablation (*bottom, arrow*). (*Right*) Parasternal long-axis view from transthoracic echocardiography in a patient with both HCM and secondary mitral regurgitation. In this patient, there is septal hypertrophy (*top, arrow*) and systolic anterior motion of the mitral valve (*middle, arrowhead*). The jet of mitral regurgitation is posterior and thus secondary to the LVOT obstruction. Ao, ascending aorta; LA, left atrium; LV, left ventricle; RV, right ventricle; VS, ventricular septum; *, ventricular septum. (*From* Sorajja P, Structural Heart Cases: A Color Atlas of Pearls and Pitfalls (2018).)

bundle branch, whose block occurs in ∼50% of cases.[5] Thus, for patients with baseline abnormalities of left bundle branch block, severe left axis deviation, or a wide QRS interval, the rate of pacemaker dependency with ASA is ∼50%. However, pacemaker dependency from complete atrioventricular block still occurs in ∼10% of patients with a normal electrocardiogram.

The authors' favored approach has been to use activation fixation leads, which are safe for indwelling during patient movement. Importantly, the temporary pacemaker lead should be implanted remote from the target site of ablation to ensure continuous capture during the septal infarction and associated edema.

Procedural Hemodynamics

Although Doppler echocardiography is highly accurate for the calculation of the LVOT gradient in HCM, comprehensive invasive hemodynamic

> **Box 1**
> **National guidelines relevant to alcohol septal ablation**
>
> **Class I**
>
> - In patients with obstructive HCM who remain severely symptomatic despite guideline directed medical therapy (GDMT), septal reduction therapy (SRT) in eligible patients, performed at experienced centers, is recommended for relieving left ventricular outflow tract obstruction (LVOTO), level of evidence ((LOE), B-non-randomized (B-NR)
>
> - In symptomatic patients with obstructive HCM who have associated cardiac disease requiring surgical treatment (eg, associated anomalous papillary muscle, markedly elongated anterior mitral leaflet, intrinsic mitral valve disease, multivessel coronary artery disease (CAD), valvular aortic stenosis), surgical myectomy, performed at experienced centers, is recommended (LOE, B-NR)
>
> - In adult patients with obstructive HCM who remain severely symptomatic, despite GDMT and in whom surgery is contraindicated or the risk is considered unacceptable because of serious comorbidities or advanced age, alcohol septal ablation in eligible patients, performed at experienced centers, is recommended (LOE, C-LD).
>
> **Class IIb**
>
> - In patients with obstructive HCM, earlier new york heart assocation ((NYHA) class II) surgical myectomy performed at comprehensive HCM centers may be reasonable in the presence of additional clinical factors, including (LOE, B-NR):
>
>   a. Severe and progressive pulmonary hypertension thought to be attributable to LVOTO or associated mitral regurgitation (MR);
>
>   b. Left atrial enlargement with 1 or more episodes of symptomatic atrial fibrillation (AF);
>
>   c. Poor functional capacity attributable to LVOTO as documented on treadmill exercise testing;
>
>   d. Children and young adults with very high resting LVOT gradients (>100 mm Hg).
>
> - For severely symptomatic patients with obstructive HCM, SRT in eligible patients, performed at experienced centers, may be considered as an alternative to escalation of medical therapy after shared decision making including risks and benefits of all treatment options (LOE, C-LD)

> **Class III: HARM**
>
> - For patients with HCM who are asymptomatic and have normal exercise capacity, SRT is not recommended (LOE, C-LD)

studies should be performed in all patients during ASA. These studies determine the acute effectiveness, which not only guides the procedure but also is a strong predictor of the long-term clinical outcomes.[6]

The operator should be cognizant of the sensitivity of LVOT obstruction to loading conditions and contractility when examining hemodynamic data from both echocardiography and catheterization. Attention must be given not only to the LVOT gradients at rest but all dynamic gradients observed during the procedure (eg, post-ventricular contraction (PVC) accentuation, variation with respiration, change with Valsalva maneuver or amyl nitrate inhalation). Of note, even mild variation in intrathoracic pressure during quiet respiration can result in large changes in LVOT obstruction (Fig. 2).

Transseptal catheterization is the most accurate method for the invasive evaluation of LVOT obstruction in HCM. In this approach, a balloon-tipped catheter with side holes (eg, 7F Berman catheter, Arrow International Inc, Reading, PA, USA) and filled with carbon dioxide can be positioned at the left ventricular inflow region. A pigtail catheter is placed retrograde in the ascending aorta for simultaneous sampling for the LVOT gradient. The transseptal approach helps to avoid catheter entrapment, which can be difficult to distinguish from changes in left ventricular pressure that occur due to the highly dynamic nature of LVOT obstruction. Use of a sheath with a sidearm port (eg, 8F Mullins) for the transseptal access also enables simultaneous recording of left atrial pressure for assessment for concomitant diastolic dysfunction and the impact of mitral regurgitation (Fig. 3).

If left ventricular pressure is assessed retrograde across the aortic valve, a pigtail catheter with shaft side holes should not be used because these holes will be positioned above the level of subaortic obstruction, leading to erroneous measurements of ventricular pressure and the LVOT gradient. Catheters that may be used for this purpose are a multipurpose with side holes at the catheter tip or a Halo pigtail. Single end-hole catheters (eg, Judkins right) are not recommended due to the tendency for entrapment. Absence of catheter entrapment should

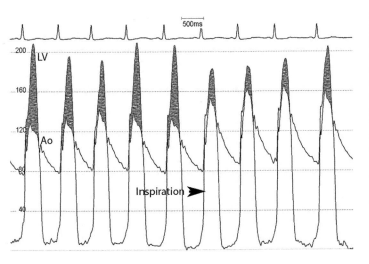

Fig. 2. Reversed pulsus paradoxus. Reversed pulsus paradoxus occurs in patients with obstructive HCM and needs to be distinguished from cardiac tamponade. These graphs show simultaneous assessment of ascending aortic and left ventricular pressures in a patient with obstructive HCM. Note the dynamic nature of the LVOT gradient even during quiet respiration. During expiration, positive thoracic pressure leads to a decrease in afterload, followed by increases in the LVOT gradient. Conversely, inspiration augments afterload, and thereby decreases LVOT obstruction, followed by an increase in the aortic pulse pressure. These changes are not mediated by preload alterations. In cardiac tamponade, there is pulsus paradoxus, which is indicated by an inspiratory decrease in the aortic pulse pressure. The expiratory and inspiratory phases of respiration in these patients are indicated by the changes in ventricular diastolic pressure or atrial pressures. (*From* Sorajja P, Structural Heart Cases: A Color Atlas of Pearls and Pitfalls (2018).)

be confirmed with examination of pressure waveforms, hand contrast injections, or demonstration of pulsatile flow with disconnection from the tube extenders used for pressure transduction.

Coronary Angiography

As stated previously, both the left and right coronary arteries should be studied, because basal septal branches occasionally arise from the proximal right coronary artery. The use of straight and caudal right anterior oblique views helps to examine the angulation of the origin of the septal artery, whereas cranial projections can assist with vessel length. The course of the artery in the ventricular septum should be confirmed in the left anterior oblique projections. Although the length of the septal artery may not be entirely visible on angiography and appear short, the vessel often can still be wired distally for support. Thus, the most important factors for choosing a septal perforator artery are location (ie, proximity to myocardial area targeted

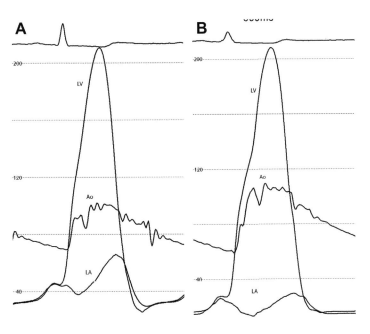

Fig. 3. Invasive hemodynamics in hypertrophic cardiomyopathy. Simultaneous recording of left atrial (LA) pressure can be beneficial because the LA pressure may vary despite the presence of severe LVOT obstruction. (*A*) Severe LVOT obstruction with high LA pressure. (*B*) Severe LVOT obstruction with normal LA pressure.

for ablation), proximal width, and angulation, rather than vessel length.

Alcohol Septal Ablation

Standard procedural anticoagulation (eg, heparin 70–100 units/kg) is given. Large (ie, 7F) guide catheters should be used to facilitate high-quality contrast injections that ensure no communication between the septal artery and epicardia vessel during balloon occlusion. A primary and a large secondary bend matched to the size of the left anterior descending (LAD) should be created at the tip of a standard-length 0.014 in guidewire to facilitate entry into the septal artery. The wire is loaded into a slightly oversized, (eg, 2.0-mm balloon for a 1.5-mm vessel), short-length (eg, 9 mm), over-the-wire balloon. The wire is carried distal to ensure the stiff portion is at the occlusion site, helping to facilitate balloon delivery and minimize balloon movement during the procedure. Oversizing of the balloon is important because it allows occlusion of the septal artery at low pressures (3–4 atm), which permits easy injection of material through the wire lumen of the catheter with minimal risk of septal artery dissection or trauma. The guidewire is withdrawn following inflation of the balloon catheter.

Coronary angiography is performed to demonstrate no communication between the septal perforator and left anterior descending artery during balloon inflation in the right anterior oblique view, and then repeated to confirm the course of the balloon in the target vessel through the ventricular septum in the left anterior oblique view. Using undiluted contrast, septal artery angiography through the balloon catheter confirms patency of the vessel for ablation and localization (ie, no untoward collateralization). During all septal injections, care should be taken because excessive force can result in vessel dissection and opening of distal collaterals. Angiographic contrast can be visible on echocardiography for identification of the perfusion bed, although many operators prefer to additionally inject echocardiographic contrast (eg, 0.5 mL Definity or Optison) (Fig. 4). Multiple echocardiographic views are used to confirm enhancement of the septal hypertrophy related to LVOT obstruction and the absence of undesirable locations, such as the areas of the septum more distal or proximal to the target region, ventricular free walls, right ventricle, or papillary muscles (Fig. 5). After identification of the targeted myocardium, desiccated ethanol is infused slowly over a period of 3 to 5 minutes followed by ~1.0 mL slow normal saline flush

to eliminate any remaining alcohol in the balloon catheter lumen. In general, the dose of alcohol is 0.8 mL per 10 mm of septal wall thickness with a maximal limit of 2.5 mL, and the authors strongly prefer less than 2 mL. The use of alcohol immediately results in a discrete myocardial infarction. In other percutaneous methods (eg, vascular coiling, covered stent placement), septal infarction may not result due to septal collateralization that is either preexisting or develops during follow-up.

The balloon should be left inflated following saline flush for greater than 5 minutes to reduce the likelihood of alcohol extravasation into the epicardial vessel. For patient comfort, intravenous sedation or analgesia (eg, fentanyl, 25–50 mg) frequently is given prophylactically or as needed. Other septal perforator arteries can be targeted and treated in a similar fashion when there is not significant reduction of either the resting or provoked LVOT gradient. Notably, the residual LVOT gradient is a strong predictor of poor clinical outcome in patients who undergo ASA.[6] When assessing the acute result of the procedure, it is important to repeat hemodynamic evaluation with large-lumen catheters devoid of the ablation equipment, because the balloon catheters will lead to pressure dampening. The LVOT gradient should also be assessed at rest and after provocative maneuvers (eg, postectopic accentuation). In general, residual peak gradients less than 30 mm Hg and preferably less than 10 mm Hg are desired, prompting termination of the procedure.

CLINICAL OUTCOMES

Acute Procedural Success

Overall, ASA typically results in an 80% reduction in the LVOT gradient. Acute results similar to surgery with a final residual resting gradient of less than or equal to 10 mm Hg occurs in 80% to 85% of patients.[6,7] Factors associated with higher likelihood of acute hemodynamic success include relatively less septal hypertrophy, lower LVOT gradients, and greater operator experience.[8] It is important to note that myocardial edema from the infarction can lead to recurrent LVOT obstruction in the subacute period and can be a source of confusion regarding the acute effect of the procedure, but that this edema subsides with ventricular remodeling. Ventricular remodeling and basal septal thinning leads to further reduction in the LVOT gradient in follow-up with maximal effects evident by 6 months. Of note, regression of myocardial hypertrophy at the site of LVOT

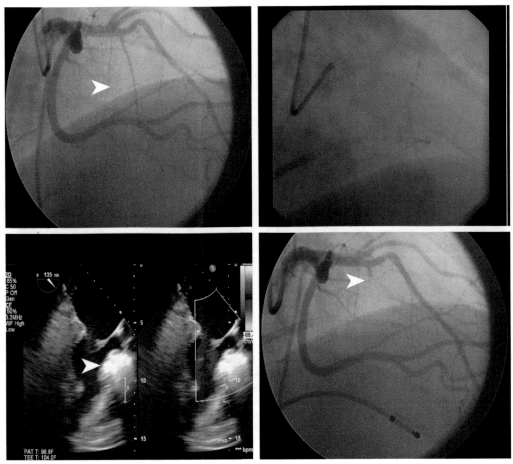

Fig. 4. Alcohol septal ablation. (*Top left*) Coronary angiography identifies the candidate septal artery (*arrowhead*). (*Top right*) An over-the-wire balloon is inserted followed by inflation and septal angiography. Echocardiographic contrast is then administered. (*Bottom left*) Comprehensive echocardiography confirms the location of the perfusion bed to be related to LVOT obstruction (*arrowhead*), and no other locations. (*Bottom right*) Following alcohol infusion, septal angiography confirms thrombosis of the vessel and territory (*arrowhead*).

obstruction from the infarction and also remotely from the ventricular septum has been demonstrated in studies using cardiac MRI, and may be responsible for improved diastolic function and further reductions in symptoms.[9]

Procedural failure most frequently results from the lack of an appropriate septal artery, which may be absent in up to 20% of patients.[10] The most common complication of ASA is temporary or complete atrioventricular block. Conduction abnormalities usually present during the procedure, but can occur subacutely due to myocardial edema from infarction; late heart block is rare. Other potential complications (<1%) are cardiac tamponade, ventricular arrhythmia, dissection of the left anterior descending artery, ventricular septal defect, and free wall myocardial infarction. Overall, periprocedural mortality for ASA is 1% to 2%.

Symptom Improvement

The clinical effectiveness of ASA has been demonstrated with improvements in both New York Heart Association functional class and objective testing, such as treadmill exercise time and peak exercise myocardial oxygen consumption. The clinical effectiveness of ASA is related to the degree of reduction in severity of the LVOT gradient. Overall, ASA typically results in a ~25% increase in objective measures of functional capacity.

Repeat procedures occasionally may be required (~5% of cases). Shadowing of the basal septum from echocardiographic contrast can occur with imaging from the transthoracic apical windows, leading to the false impression of successful ablation of the most proximal portion and resulting in residual obstructive hypertrophy. Stunning of the ventricular septum from

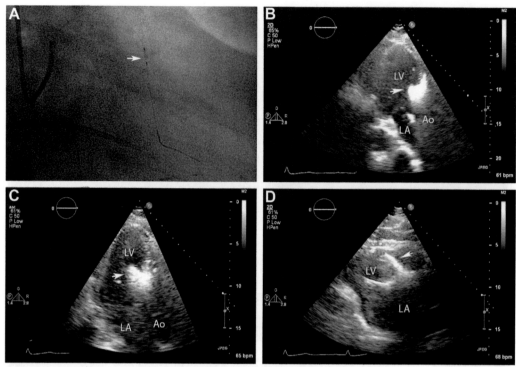

Fig. 5. Contrast enhancement of papillary muscles (*A, arrows*) in a patient with hypertrophic cardiomyopathy during an attempt at alcohol septal ablation. (*A*) The most proximal septal perforator artery is wired with a standard 0.014 in. soft-tip guidewire, followed by placement and inflation of a 1.5-mm over-the-wire angioplasty balloon to 3 atm. The guidewire is then removed. (*B*) Through the angioplasty balloon, echocardiographic contrast (Definity) is injected with simultaneous transthoracic echocardiography. Echocardiography demonstrates contrast enhancement of ventricular septal myocardium that is intimately involved in the creation of systolic anterior of the mitral valve and left ventricular outflow tract obstruction (*arrow*). (*C*) With further imaging, however, there also is contrast enhancement of the inferomedial papillary muscle (*arrow*). (*D*) Additional imaging demonstrates contrast enhancement of the entire inferomedial papillary muscle extending toward the left ventricular free wall (*arrow*). Given the potential for papillary muscle infarction, the alcohol septal ablation procedure was then aborted. Ao, ascending aorta; LA, left atrium; LV, left ventricle. (*From* Sorajja P, Structural Heart Cases: A Color Atlas of Pearls and Pitfalls (2018).)

balloon occlusion may occur without complete infarction, leading to recovery of septal function and recurrent LVOT obstruction in follow-up. Although several studies have shown clinical improvements comparable to that of myectomy, symptom relief may be greater with surgery in younger patients (Fig. 6). The reasons for this observation are not clear, but may be related to the residual gradients present after ablation (typically 10–20 mm Hg) that are consequently higher than those after surgical myectomy (typically <10 mm Hg). These relatively higher residual gradients may be less tolerated by younger, more active individuals.

Survival

Several single-center studies have compared the results of ASA with those of surgical myectomy with follow-up extending 8 to 10 years.[6,7,11–20] Overall survival has been comparable to that of surgery in several series, although the total number of patients in these comparative analyses remains relatively small. One notable exception is a study of 91 patients treated at Erasmus MC Rotterdam that raised concern regarding potential for arrhythmias after ablation. The study was noteworthy for a relatively higher average alcohol dose (3.5 ± 1.5 mL) among their patients, including a mean dose of 4.5 ± 1.2 mL in the first 25 patients. In other studies, in which long-term survival was not impaired, the mean alcohol dose was only 1.8 mL, and the septal wall thickness was similar to that of the patients in the Rotterdam study (23 ± 5 mm vs 23 ± 5 mm). Of note, early studies of ASA, in which contrast

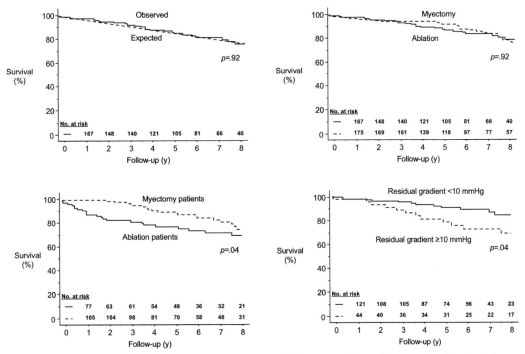

Fig. 6. Survival free of death or severe symptoms in patients with hypertrophic cardiomyopathy after alcohol septal ablation. (*Top left*) Observed survival for the patients undergoing ablation versus expected survival, which was calculated using US population death rates for year of entry into study, age, and gender. (*Bottom left*) Comparison of survival free of all-cause mortality for the patients undergoing ablation versus survival of age- and sex-matched patients undergoing myectomy. (*Top right*) For patients younger than 65 years, survival free of all-cause mortality and severe symptoms was better for patients undergoing surgery than the patients undergoing ablation. (*Bottom right*) Survival free of all-cause mortality for the patients undergoing ablation according to residual left ventricular outflow tract gradient. (Reproduced with permission from Sorajja et al.[6])

echocardiography was not routinely performed, were associated with larger infarct size, a greater risk of complications, and poorer clinical outcome.[21]

In a multicenter registry of 874 patients undergoing alcohol ablation that included patients from aforementioned studies, there was significant improvement in functional status (~5% with residual severe symptoms). Overall survival was 74% at 9 years of follow-up with predictors of death being lower baseline ejection fraction, fewer arteries treated, larger number of ablation procedures, and higher septal thickness postablation.[22] Several large-scale registries and meta-analyses have examined the outcome of patients undergoing ASA when compared with surgery.[23–25] Taken together, the aforementioned studies suggest that efficacious and comparable outcomes can be achieved with appropriate patient selection, use of lower doses of alcohol, and greater operator and institutional experience in the comprehensive care of patients with HCM.

PERSPECTIVES FOR THE CLINICIAN

Although septal ablation is effective in selected patients with HCM, its introduction has been met with concerns due to the safety and durable results of surgery, potential procedural morbidity of septal ablation (eg, pacemaker dependency), and possible long-term deleterious effects of the therapeutic infarction. The selection of either ASA or surgery will continue to rely on expert consensus, because randomized clinical trials in this field have been deemed to be not feasible.[26] For some patients, ASA may be the only option for definitive relief of LVOT obstruction due to poor candidacy for surgery. In others, ASA can be offered after the risks of the procedure and the aforementioned concerns have been discussed fully with the patient. Without the need for general anesthesia and open surgery, the relatively less invasive aspects of ASA are its principal advantages. Hospital stay (typically 3–5 days) and physical rehabilitation is also relatively shorter. These issues are particularly relevant for elderly patients or those with morbidities that significantly increase the risk of open surgical repair. Of note, among patients who underwent septal ablation in one study, 20% of these patients were believed to be at significantly increased operative risk for myectomy due to patient age (≥75 years) or presence of severe comorbidities (eg, end-stage renal disease, porcelain aorta, morbid obesity, cor pulmonale).[7]

Importantly, even though ASA uses conventional coronary angioplasty equipment, the procedure is complex with a steep learning curve and unique complications.[8] Recent data have highlighted the beneficial effects of ASA for relatively younger patients, although a balanced discussion must still be undertaken when counseling patients.[27,28] In addition, patients with HCM are uniquely complex in terms of diagnosis and management, with many factors that should be taken into account when considering septal reduction therapy. Thus, national guidelines recommend that these management considerations be made in a tertiary center, where expertise in both percutaneous and surgical options can be offered.[3]

CLINICS CARE POINTS

- When evaluating a patient with severely symptomatic, obstructive HCM, consider referral to a center of expertise for septal reduction therapy.

- For determining candidacy for ASA, focus on identifying the mechanism of LVOT obstruction as being dynamic, and related to systolic anterior motion of the mitral valve, in the absence of intrinsic mitral valve disease.

REFERENCES

1. Sigwart U. Non-surgical myocardial reduction for hypertrophic obstructive cardiomyopathy. Lancet 1995;346:211–4.

2. Ommen SR, Maron BJ, Olivotto I, et al. Long-term effects of surgical myectomy on survival in patients with obstructive hypertrophic cardiomyopathy. J Am Coll Cardiol 2005;46:470–6.

3. Ommen SR, Mital S, Burke MA, et al. 2020 AHA/ACC guideline for the diagnosis and treatment of patients with hypertrophic cardiomyopathy: executive summary: a report of the american college of cardiology/american heart association joint committee on clinical practice guidelines. Circulation 2020;142(25):e533–57.

4. Valeti US, Nishimura RA, Holmes DR, et al. Comparison of surgical septal myectomy and alcohol septal ablation with cardiac magnetic resonance imaging in patients with hypertrophic obstructive cardiomyopathy. J Am Coll Cardiol 2007;49:350–7.

5. Talreja DR, Nishimura RA, Edwards WD, et al. Alcohol septal ablation versus surgical septal myectomy: comparison of effects on atrioventricular conduction tissue. J Am Coll Cardiol 2004;44:2329–32.

6. Sorajja P, Ommen SR, Holmes DR Jr, et al. Survival after alcohol septal ablation for obstructive hypertrophic cardiomyopathy. Circulation 2012;126:2374–80.

7. Sorajja P, Valeti U, Nishimura RA, et al. Outcome of alcohol septal ablation for obstructive hypertrophic cardiomyopathy. Circulation 2008;118:131–9.

8. Sorajja P, Binder J, Nishimura RA, et al. Predictors of an optimal clinical outcome with alcohol septal ablation for obstructive hypertrophic cardiomyopathy. Catheter Cardiovasc Interv 2013;81:E58–67.

9. Van Dockum WG, Beek AM, ten Cate FJ, et al. Early onset and progression of left ventricular remodeling after alcohol septal ablation in hypertrophic obstructive cardiomyopathy. Circulation 2005;111:2503–8.

10. Singh M, Edwards WD, Holmes DR Jr, et al. Anatomy of the first septal perforating artery: a study with implications for ablation therapy for hypertrophic cardiomyopathy. Mayo Clin Proc 2001;76:799–802.

11. Firoozi S, Elliott PM, Sharma S, et al. Septal myotomy-myectomy and transcoronary septal alcohol ablation in hypertrophic obstructive cardiomyopathy: a comparison of clinical, hemodynamic and exercise outcomes. Eur Heart J 2002;23:1617–24.

12. Nagueh S, Ommen SR, Lakkis NM, et al. Comparison of ethanol septal reduction therapy with surgical myectomy for the treatment of hypertrophic obstructive cardiomyopathy. J Am Coll Cardiol 2001;38:1701–6.

13. Qin JX, Shiota T, Lever HM, et al. Outcome of patients with hypertrophic obstructive cardiomyopathy after percutaneous transluminal septal myocardial ablation and septal myectomy surgery. J Am Coll Cardiol 2001;38:1994–2000.

14. Ralph-Edwards A, Woo A, McCrindle BW, et al. Hypertrophic obstructive cardiomyopathy: comparison of outcomes after myectomy or alcohol ablation adjusted by propensity score. J Thorac Cardiovasc Surg 2005;129:351–8.

15. Jiang TY, Wu XS, Lu Q, et al. Transcoronary ablation of septal hypertrophy compared with surgery in the treatment of hypertrophic obstructive cardiomyopathy. Chin Med J 2004;117:296–8.

16. Vural AH, Tiryakioglu O, Turk T, et al. Treatment modalities in hypertrophic obstructive cardiomyopathy: surgical myectomy versus percutaneous septal ablation. Heart Surg Forum 2007;10:493–7.

17. Fernandes VL, Nielsen C, Nagueh SF, et al. Follow-up of alcohol septal ablation for symptomatic hypertrophic obstructive cardiomyopathy: the Baylor and Medical University of South Carolina experience 1996 to 2007. JACC Cardiovasc Interv 2008;1:561–70.

18. Kwon DH, Kapadia SR, Tuzcu EM, et al. Long-term outcomes in high-risk symptomatic patients with hypertrophic cardiomyopathy undergoing alcohol septal ablation. JACC Cardiovasc Interv 2008;1:432–8.

19. Vriesendorp PA, Liebregts M, Steggerda RC, et al. Long-term outcomes after medical and invasive treatment in patients with hypertrophic cardiomyopathy. JACC Heart Fail 2014;2:630–6.

20. Ten Cate FJ, Solimon OI, Michels M, et al. Long-term outcome of alcohol septal ablation in patients with obstructive hypertrophic cardiomyopathy: a word of caution. Circ Heart Fail 2010;3:362–9.

21. Faber L, Seggewiss Gleichman U. Percutaneous transluminal septal myocardial ablation in hypertrophic obstructive cardiomyopathy. Results with respect to intraprocedural myocardial contrast echocardiography. Circulation 1998;98:2415–21.

22. Nagueh SF, Groves BM, Schwartz L, et al. Alcohol septal ablation for the treatment of hypertrophic obstructive cardiomyopathy. A multicenter North American registry. J Am Coll Cardiol 2011;58: 2322–8.

23. Agarwal S, Tuzcu EM, Desai MY, et al. Updated meta-analysis of septal alcohol ablation versus myectomy for hypertrophic cardiomyopathy. J Am Coll Cardiol 2010;55:823–34.

24. Alam M, Doakinsih H, Lakkis NM. Hypertrophic obstructive cardiomyopathy- alcohol septal ablation vs. myectomy: a meta-analysis. Eur Heart J 2009;30:1080–7.

25. Veselka J, Faber L, Liebregts M, et al. Outcome of alcohol septal ablation in mildly symptomatic patients with hypertrophic obstructive cardiomyopathy: a long-term follow-up study based on the euro-alcohol septal ablation registry. J Am Heart Assoc 2017;6(5):e005735. pii.

26. Olivotto I, Ommen SR, Maron MS, et al. Surgical myectomy versus alcohol septal ablation for obstructive hypertrophic cardiomyopathy. Will there ever be a randomized trial. J Am Coll Cardiol 2007;50:831–4.

27. Liebregts M, Faber L, Jensen MK, et al. Outcomes of alcohol septal ablation in younger patients with obstructive hypertrophic cardiomyopathy. JACC Cardiovasc Interv 2017;10:1134–43.

28. Sorajja P. Alcohol septal ablation for obstructive hypertrophic cardiomyopathy: a word of balance. J Am Coll Cardiol 2017;70:489–94.

Use of Electrosurgery in Interventional Cardiology

Jaffar M. Khan, BM BCh, PhD[a], Toby Rogers, BM BCh, PhD[a,b],
Adam B. Greenbaum, MD[c], Vasilis C. Babaliaros, MD[c],
Christopher G. Bruce, MB ChB[a], Robert J. Lederman, MD[a,*]

KEYWORDS

- Basilica • Lampoon • TAVR • TMVR

KEY POINTS

- Transcatheter Electrosurgery enables precise tissue traversal and laceration through charge concentration at the target tissue.
- BASILICA mitigates coronary artery obstruction from TAVR in native or bioprosthetic valves.
- LAMPOON mitigates LVOT obstruction from TMVR, particularly when using valves with an open-cell design.
- ELASTA-Clip enables TMVR after TEER by liberating the device from the anterior mitral leaflet.

BACKGROUND

Transcatheter electrosurgery is a versatile tool that can be used to cut cardiac tissue without the need for a sternotomy, cardiopulmonary bypass, and cardioplegia. In fact, a controlled laceration can be performed using off-the-shelf equipment through 2 vascular sheaths and under local anesthesia. With adequate imaging and suitable anatomy, any cardiac tissue can be cut. Thus, transcatheter electrosurgery can provide bespoke therapies for complex patients who often have no other good treatment options.

In this review, we will discuss the common applications for electrosurgical tissue traversal and laceration, summarizing the evidence and the key technical steps for each.

PRINCIPLES OF TRANSCATHETER ELECTROSURGERY

Alternating current at radiofrequencies is transmitted through a guidewire to the target tissue, whereby it concentrates and generates heat. The water inside cells boils when it reaches 100 °C and the cells vaporize. This, in essence, is tissue "cutting." The effects on tissue of different heating thresholds are shown in Table 1.

From a practical standpoint, effective insulation is necessary to ensure sufficient charge concentration at the target tissue to effect cutting, and prevent unwanted dispersal in adjacent tissues including blood, which may coagulate and cause guidewire charring. Insulation is achieved by careful positioning of insulating microcatheters and guiding catheters, selectively denuding the guidewire polytetrafluoroethylene (PTFE) coating at the electrical contact points, and dispersing blood with nonionic 5% dextrose solution.

EQUIPMENT

Dedicated equipment for "traversal-only" transcatheter electrosurgery applications that are currently marketed include the VersaCross wire

---

[a] Cardiovascular Branch, Division of Intramural Research, National Heart Lung and Blood Institute, National Institutes of Health, Building 10, Room 2c713, MSC 1538, Bethesda, MD 20892-1538, USA; [b] Medstar Washington Hospital Center, 110 Irving Street, Northwest, Washington, DC 20010, USA; [c] Structural Heart and Valve Center, Emory University Hospital, 550 Peachtree Street Northeast, Medical Office Tower, Fl 6, Atlanta, GA 30308, USA
* Corresponding author. Cardiovascular Branch, Division of Intramural Research, National Heart Lung and Blood Institute, National Institutes of Health, Building 10, Room 2c713, MSC 1538, Bethesda, MD 20892-1538.
E-mail address: lederman@nih.gov
Twitter: @CathElectroSurg (J.M.K.); @AdamGreenbaumMD (A.B.G.); @ChrisGBruce13 (C.G.B.); @TheBethesda-Labs (R.J.L.)

Table 1
Tissue effects at rising temperatures

Temperature	Tissue Effect
49° C	Tissue coagulates
60° C	Protein denatures
70° C	Cells desiccate
100° C	Cells rupture from the vaporization of intracellular water

Adapted from Pearce JA. Electrosurgery. 1 ed. New York: Wiley Medical, 1986.

and the NRG needle for transseptal access, and the PowerWire RF guidewire and Nykanen RF wire for peripheral intervention (Baylis Medical, Austin, TX).

Coronary guidewires may be used off-label, with minor benchtop modifications, for both electrosurgical tissue traversal as well as laceration. Guidewires that perform best have a high tip load, a core-to-tip design, and a wire tip without a polymer jacket[1]. We typically use the Astato XS 20 300cm guidewire (Asahi Intecc, Japan) for most of our transcatheter electrosurgery procedures. The distal PTFE coating is stripped with a scalpel at the point whereby the guidewire is connected to an electrosurgery pencil and generator with hemostatic forceps.

For traversal, the entire length of the guidewire inside the body is insulated in a microcatheter, typically a locking Piggyback Wire Converter (Teleflex, NC), with only the guidewire tip exposed. Once the tip is in contact with the target tissue, the guidewire is advanced through the microcatheter and perforates through the tissue during brief electrification at 30 to 50W continuous duty cycle "pure cut" mode.

For laceration, the microcatheter is withdrawn to the proximal half of the guidewire. The midshaft of the guidewire, adjacent to the Piggyback tip, is selectively denuded along 4mm of the guidewire length and across a 90° arc with the blade of a scalpel. The blunt end of the scalpel acts as a pivot to kink the denuded segment in the middle. The result is selective inner curvature denudation that will direct the current onto the target tissue and is called the flying V. The flying V is positioned across the target tissue between 2 guiding catheters which direct the laceration. 5% dextrose is infused during laceration to displace blood during current application. This serves 2 purposes. First, it displaces blood, preventing coagulation and

thromboembolism, and char formation on the guidewire. Second, it is nonionic and so acts as an extra-insulator, concentrating charge dispersal at the target tissue.

ELECTROSURGERY TO RECANALIZE OCCLUSIVE LESIONS

The first reported use of transcatheter electrosurgery was to restore right ventricular to pulmonary artery flow in patients with atretic pulmonary valves[2]. The atretic tissue is traversed with a guidewire during brief application of radiofrequency energy.

The technique has been used to recanalize central and peripheral vascular occlusions. Particularly pertinent to the interventional cardiologist, transcatheter electrosurgery has also been reported to recanalize an ostial right coronary artery chronic total occlusion when re-entry was not feasible using tapered stiff guidewires[3]. In this report, a Confianza guidewire (Asahi), insulated in a Piggyback microcatheter, was briefly electrified to achieve successful luminal re-entry.

TRANSSEPTAL PUNCTURE

Perhaps the commonest application of electrosurgery in interventional cardiology is for transseptal puncture for left atrial access. By vaporizing a target on the fossa ovalis, the interatrial septum can be traversed without mechanical force, which may cause sliding of the needle and imprecise puncture or atrial back wall injury from forced advancement of the needle.

Electrosurgery-assisted transseptal puncture may be performed by electrifying a transseptal needle, electrifying a coronary guidewire, or using dedicated devices[4].

Radiofrequency access was found to be superior to needle transseptal puncture in a randomized trial, with reduced procedure time, reduced procedure failure, and reduced plastic particulate matter with the radiofrequency system (NRG Transseptal needle, Baylis)[5].

TRANSCAVAL ACCESS
Clinical need
Large bore arterial access may be required for transcatheter aortic valve replacement (TAVR), transcatheter endovascular aortic repair (TEVAR), or mechanical circulatory support. Large bore femoral arterial access is not feasible due to diseased iliofemoral arteries in 4.7% of all patients undergoing TAVR[6] and up to 30% of patients undergoing TEVAR[7].

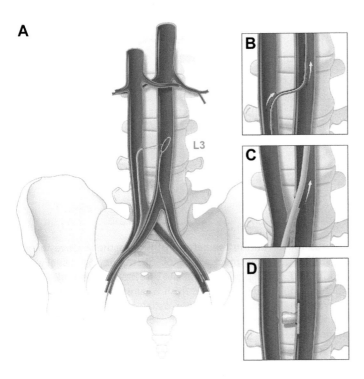

Fig. 1. Transcaval access. (A) An electrified guidewire traverses from a guide in the IVC to a snare in the infra-renal aorta. (B) Sequential microcatheters are advanced into the aorta during snare countertraction. (C) The large sheath is introduced. (D) The aortotomy is closed with a nitinol mesh device.

Transcaval access provides an ergonomic, completely percutaneous transfemoral venous access to the infrarenal aorta which can be performed under local anesthesia and moderate sedation.

Procedure technique

Preprocedure computed tomography (CT) scanning is required to assess suitability for transcaval access.[8] This typically requires a calcium-free window for traversal in the right infrarenal aortic wall, facing the inferior vena cava (IVC), and a suitable landing zone for a covered stent if bailout is needed. Orthogonal projection angles for transcaval crossing are derived and cranio-caudal height of crossing is mapped onto the lumbar vertebrae for easy reference[9].

Femoral venous access is obtained to deliver an internal mammary-shaped guide catheter (Fig. 1). Femoral arterial access is obtained to deliver a JR4 guide catheter and Gooseneck snare into the infrarenal aorta. An Astato guidewire sheathed in Piggyback and NaviCross (Terumo, NJ) microcatheters is advanced through the venous guide to the preselected crossing level and directed toward the snare. During brief electrification at 50W, the Astato guidewire is advanced through the IVC and aortic walls into the snare. The guidewire is snared and advanced up toward the aortic arch. With snare countertraction on the guidewire, the Piggyback and

NaviCross microcatheters are sequentially advanced into the aorta. The Piggyback and Astato guidewire are then exchanged for a stiff 0.035" Lunderquist guidewire (Cook Medical, IN) through the NaviCross microcatheter. A large-bore vascular sheath is advanced over the Lunderquist guidewire securing central arterial access.

Access port closure is attempted after full reversal of heparin with protamine. A pigtail catheter in the aorta marks the transcaval crossing site. A 10/8 Amplatzer Duct Occluder (ADO, Abbott, IL) in an Agilis small curl deflectable sheath (Abbott) is advanced through the transcaval access sheath alongside a 0.014" safety buddy wire. The transcaval sheath is briskly withdrawn all the way back into the IVC. The aortic disc of the ADO is exposed in the aorta. The system is withdrawn and the deflectable sheath is flexed to position the aortic disc flush against the aortic wall at the transcaval access site. While maintaining gentle tension on the ADO cable, the deflectable sheath is withdrawn and unflexed to expose the body of the ADO device. Aortography is performed to confirm adequate device position and the ADO is released. Final cineangiography is performed and closure assessed. In rare cases of retroperitoneal extravasation, balloon aortic tamponade should be performed, followed by covered stent deployment if needed.

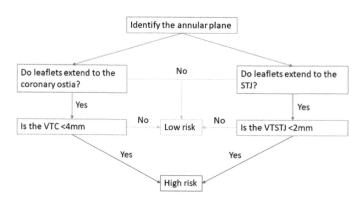

Fig. 2. Algorithm for predicting coronary obstruction.

In cases of emergency transcaval access for mechanical circulatory support, some modifications to this procedure may be required. In lieu of a preprocedure CT, 2 pigtail catheters, in the IVC and infrarenal aorta, are aligned in orthogonal projections to determine the optimal transcaval crossing fluoroscopic projection angles. A 24F >33cm sheath is inserted to accommodate a 5.0 Impella device (Abiomed, MA). On removal, the transcaval sheath is thoroughly aspirated for clot. The same sequence for closure is followed as above but a 12/10 ADO is used for closure due to access and increased sheath size.

Clinical evidence

In the prospective 100 patient NHLBI Transcaval TAVR trial, transcaval access was successful in 99% of subjects, inpatient survival was 96%, and the rate of life-threatening bleeding was 7%.[10] The median hospital stay was 4 days in this early experience. There was no late bleeding associated with transcaval tracts at 1 year[11].

TEVAR has been successfully performed via transcaval access, which provides an attractive percutaneous alternative in patients with diseased iliofemoral arteries[12].

Transcaval access is feasible for emergency percutaneous implantation of a 7mm Impella 5.0 mechanical circulatory support device.[13] In a single-center series, 10 patients with progressive or refractive cardiogenic shock underwent Impella 5.0 device implantation via transcaval access without preprocedural CT guidance. Six patients survived to access port closure and discharge.

BASILICA

Clinical need

TAVR causes coronary obstruction in about 1% of all cases, with a 40% to 50% mortality[14]. It is commoner in patients with smaller anatomy and in the setting of bioprosthetic valve failure. The mechanism of obstruction is usually the displacement of the diseased aortic leaflet which may either lie flush against the coronary artery ostium (coronary ostial obstruction) or against the sinotubular junction (sinus sequestration).

Coronary obstruction can be predicted on preprocedure CT. The simplified algorithm we use is shown in Fig. 2.

Bioprosthetic or native Aortic Scallop Intentional Laceration to prevent Iatrogenic Coronary Artery obstruction (BASILICA) is a transcatheter electrosurgical technique to lacerate diseased aortic valve leaflets immediately before TAVR in patients at risk of coronary obstruction[15].

Procedure technique

Orthogonal fluoroscopic projection angles for the target leaflet are derived from preprocedure CT.[16] General anesthesia and TEE guidance may help with catheter positioning, troubleshooting, and early recognition of complications, but is not mandatory.

A 14F sheath with balloon inflatable hemostatic hub (Gore DrySeal Flex, Gore Medical, DE) is inserted in the femoral artery used for TAVR. If performing *solo* BASILICA, a 6F sheath is placed in the contralateral femoral artery. For *doppio* BASILICA, the contralateral sheath is upsized to a second 14F sheath.

The first step is positioning of the snare (Fig. 3). The aortic valve is crossed using standard techniques from the contralateral arterial access. A multipurpose guiding catheter is positioned in the left ventricular outflow tract (LVOT) and stabilized with a 0.018″ guidewire in the left ventricle. An appropriately sized Gooseneck snare (typically 20mm or 25mm) is positioned to circumscribe the LVOT.

The second step is positioning of the traversal system. We recommend the catheter escalation to 50W. The guidewire tip is snared in the LVOT. Care is taken not to snare below the anterior mitral valve leaflet as this risks entrapping chords that would result in chord laceration during BASILICA.

The fourth step is to create the flying V. With the guidewire tip snared, the Piggyback microcatheter is withdrawn to the proximal half of the guidewire. The mid-shaft of the guidewire adjacent to the Piggyback tip is denuded and kinked as previously described. The flying V is then inserted into the body while retrieving the snared end of the guidewire and advanced till it straddles the target aortic leaflet. The microcatheter and guiding catheter positions are secured by tightening the hemostatic hubs and locking with the help of torque devices.

The fifth step is crossing the valve through the 14F sheath, adjacent to the BASILICA catheter, to position a pigtail catheter in the left ventricle.

The sixth step is leaflet laceration. Gentle tension is applied to both limbs of the catheter-guidewire system. When all the slack has been removed, 5% dextrose is infused through the catheters and current delivered at 70W for the 1 to 2 seconds required for complete laceration. The system is disassembled and withdrawn from the body. Hemodynamic compromise is rare at this stage because of the coaptation of the split leaflet during diastole.

The final step is TAVR over a stiff guidewire introduced through the prepositioned pigtail. The 14F sheath is either replaced with a balloon-expandable TAVR sheath or simply removed if using an in-line system.

Clinical evidence

The NHLBI-sponsored BASILICA IDE trial enrolled 30 subjects who required TAVR but were at high risk of coronary artery obstruction[17]. BASILICA was successfully performed in 93%, demonstrating procedure feasibility. No patient had coronary obstruction despite a central core laboratory predicting high risk in all, demonstrating procedure efficacy. There was 1 disabling (3%) and 2 nondisabling (7%) strokes following BASILICA and TAVR. There were no late events related to BASILICA between 30 days and 1 year[18].

A 214 patient BASILICA Registry assessed procedure safety in a large number of patients, as well as feasibility in the real world[19]. BASILICA was successful in 94.4% of patients. There was no culprit coronary artery obstruction in 95.3%. At 30 days, there was 2.8% death and 2.8% stroke (0.5% disabling stroke). One year survival was 83.9%. There were no differences in

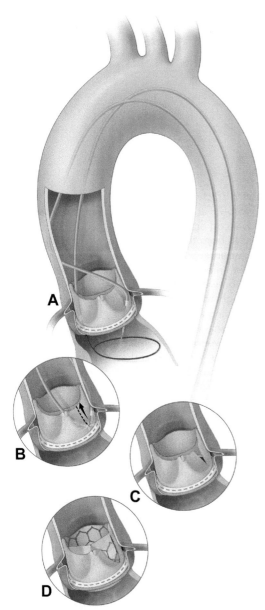

Fig. 3. BASILICA procedure steps (A) An electrified guidewire traverses from a guide in the aorta through the target aortic valve leaflet into a snare in the LVOT. (B and C) The flying V is electrified, lacerating the leaflet. (D) The leaflet splays after TAVR, maintaining coronary perfusion.

strategy outlined in Fig. 4 to obtain orthogonal traversal catheter position in the target leaflet.

The third step is to traverse the leaflet. The Astato guidewire and Piggyback microcatheter are introduced and the leaflet gently palpated with the guidewire. If the position is satisfactory, the Astato guidewire is pushed through the leaflet during brief application of current at 30

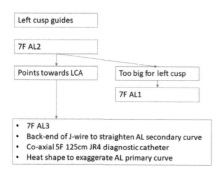

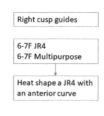

Fig. 4. Catheter escalation strategy for BASILICA.

outcomes between native and bioprosthetic valves, *solo* or *doppio* BASILICA, or in patients whereby cerebral embolic protection was used, though this was not randomized. This registry demonstrated the safety of the BASILICA procedure.

Benchtop experiments suggest BASILICA may not be suitable for all cases of TAV-in-TAV[20]. Balloon-assisted BASILICA may overcome some of these limitations[21].

BASILICA may also be used to improve TAVR implantation and expansion in bicuspid valves (Bi-SILICA).[22] Though this is feasible, the evidence to support this approach is lacking.

LAMPOON
Clinical need
LVOT obstruction is a common and often fatal complication of transcatheter mitral valve replacement (TMVR). The mitral valve prosthesis pushes the anterior mitral valve leaflet toward septum, causing *fixed* LVOT obstruction. Furthermore, the narrowed LVOT creates Bernoulli forces that may cause systolic anterior motion (SAM) of the anterior mitral valve leaflet and *dynamic* LVOT obstruction. The problem is common both when implanting TAVR valves in the mitral position, and with dedicated TMVR devices, and is a leading cause of screen failure in the early trials for these devices[23]. Preprocedure CT is key for predicting LVOT obstruction[24].

Laceration of the Anterior Mitral leaflet to Prevent Outflow Obstruction (LAMPOON) is a transcatheter electrosurgical technique performed immediately before TMVR[25,26]. The anterior leaflet is lacerated down the centerline, preserving chords, allowing the leaflet to splay away from the LVOT.

Procedure technique
The LAMPOON procedure has undergone a few iterations since conception, each with its advantages and uses in special situations[27]. We will review each in turn.

Retrograde LAMPOON
Two 6-7F JL3.5P (posterior curve) catheters are advanced either side of the anterior mitral valve leaflet from two femoral arterial sheaths.

A transseptal puncture is performed in a posterior inferior location on the fossa ovalis. A balloon-wedge end-hole catheter is floated through the major mitral valve orifice into the ascending aorta. A guidewire through this catheter is snared from the femoral artery, establishing a veno-arterial rail along a chord-free trajectory. A JL3.5P catheter is advanced over this rail into the left atrium and snare is placed. A second JL3.5P catheter is positioned at the center and base of the anterior mitral leaflet, guided by TEE. An Astato guidewire and Piggyback microcatheter are advanced to the anterior mitral leaflet through the traversal guide. The guidewire is briefly electrified at 50W and pushed through the leaflet from LVOT into the left atrium, whereby it is snared. The flying V is then formed and positioned to straddle the anterior mitral leaflet. The catheter and microcatheter positions are secured, tension is applied to both catheters and current is applied for 1–2s at 70W during a 5% dextrose infusion till the leaflet is lacerated.

The advantage of this technique is that it reproducibly creates a centerline laceration and enables prepositioning of the mitral valve prosthesis. The major drawback is difficulty positioning the traversal catheter.

Antegrade LAMPOON
Two 6F guide catheters are positioned on either side of the anterior mitral leaflet from 2 deflectable sheaths positioned across the same septostomy and femoral venous sheath[28].

Transseptal access is obtained and 2 deflectable sheaths (Agilis medium curl or similar) are positioned in the left atrium. A veno-arterial rail along a chord-free trajectory is established through one deflectable sheath as described above. A snare and JL3.5 guiding catheter is

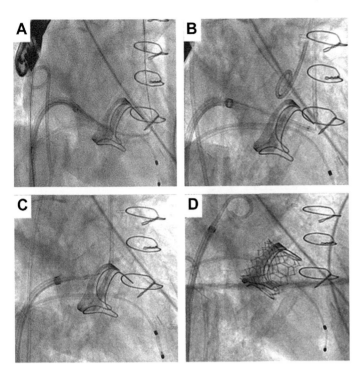

Fig. 5. Tip to Base LAMPOON (*A*). A veno-arterial rail is created through a transseptal deflectable sheath. (*B*). The flying V is positioned at the tip of the anterior leaflet of the bioprosthetic mitral valve. (*C*). The leaflet is lacerated and the flying V is stopped from further progression by the valve sewing ring. (*D*). Successful mitral valve-in-valve TMVR.

then advanced along this rail through the deflectable sheath to sit in the LVOT. A JR4 guiding catheter is advanced through the second deflectable sheath and positioned at the base of the A2 scallop of the anterior mitral leaflet. The Astato guidewire and Piggyback microcatheter are introduced and traversal proceeds from left atrium into LVOT during brief electrification at 30 to 50W. The flying V is then formed, positioned, insulated, and secured as before. Care is taken to align the laceration trajectory down the centerline by positioning the deflectable sheaths at A2. The guiding catheters are then pulled into the deflectable sheaths during laceration.

The advantage of this technique is that it provides greater stability and control for leaflet traversal. The drawback is the potential for eccentric laceration.

Tip to base and rescue LAMPOON

In the setting of a bioprosthetic mitral valve or complete ring, the traversal step can be skipped and laceration proceeds from tip to base[29]. Progression of laceration is prevented when there is a suitable "backstop."

Transseptal access is obtained with a deflectable sheath and a veno-arterial rail is created (Fig. 5). A flying V is created on the guidewire used for the rail and positioned at the tip of the anterior mitral leaflet. Tension is applied on both arterial and transseptal guiding catheters and guidewire limbs during electrification at 70W and 5% dextrose infusion. Longer and multiple burns may be required for complete laceration.

The advantage of this technique is the simplicity of the procedure. It may also be used as a rescue after TMVR when there is SAM[30]. The drawback is that it is limited to cases with a safe backstop.

Clinical evidence

The prospective NHLBI LAMPOON IDE trial investigated LAMPOON in the 30 subjects at high risk of LVOT obstruction from TMVR[31]. LAMPOON was successful in 100% of subjects, in both the setting of valve-in-ring and valve-in-mitral annular calcification. LVOT obstruction was evident in only 3% on exit from the catheter laboratory despite the prohibitive risk in all. However, subjects with a small skirt neo-LVOT[32] did require alcohol septal ablation in addition to LAMPOON, and this was later introduced as exclusion criteria to enrollment. There were no strokes and 30-day survival was 93% in this high-risk cohort.

A retrospective analysis of 21 patients who underwent tip to base LAMPOON (19 preventative, 2 rescue) demonstrated successful leaflet laceration and prevention of LVOT obstruction in all cases[33]. There were 2 cases of aortic valve

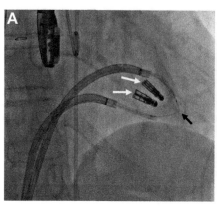
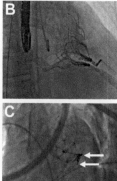

Fig. 6. ELASTA-Clip. (A). The flying V (*black arrow*) is positioned on the anterior edge of 2 MitraClip devices (*white arrows*). (B and C) The Mitra-Clip devices are secure on the posterior ventricular wall and Tendyne TMVR valve is fully expanded.

injury and both cases had a supra-annular mitral bioprosthetic ring with a small distance between the ring and the aortic valve. In summary, this technique was simple and effective, and safe in the appropriate anatomy.

ELASTA-CLIP
Clinical need

Transcatheter edge-to-edge repair (TEER) is increasingly used as a percutaneous treatment of both primary and functional mitral regurgitation. However, this therapy may prevent future TMVR. The ability to manage the TEER device using transcatheter electrosurgery is, therefore, very timely. Electrosurgical Laceration and Stabilization of Clip devices (ELASTA-Clip) is a transcatheter electrosurgical technique to create a single orifice mitral valve and enable TMVR[34].

Procedure technique

Transseptal access is obtained and 2 deflectable sheaths (Agilis medium curl or similar) are positioned across a single septostomy (Fig. 6). The deflectable sheaths direct 2 guiding catheters through the lateral and medial mitral valve orifices, respectively. A guidewire is advanced through one catheter (internal mammary-shaped guide or similar) into a snare through the second catheter (a Multipurpose shaped guide or similar). A flying V is created at the mid-shaft of the guidewire and advanced to straddle the TEER devices. The flying V is adjusted so it rests on the anterior mitral leaflet attachment to the TEER devices. Tension is applied to both catheters and guidewire limbs during brief electrification at 70W and 5% dextrose infusion. The TEER devices are liberated from the anterior leaflet while still attached to the posterior leaflet.

The ELASTA-Clip system is disassembled and TMVR is performed according to device-specific

guidelines. The TMVR device secures the clip between the cage of the valve and the posterior left ventricular wall.

Clinical evidence

A single-center series of 5 patients with mitral valve failure in the setting of previous MitraClip (Abbott) implantation underwent ELASTA-Clip and TMVR with the investigational Tendyne valve (Abbott) on a compassionate basis[35]. All patients had successful clip detachment and TMVR, and all survived to 30 days.

SUMMARY

Transcatheter electrosurgery encompasses a diverse portfolio of procedures to enable therapies in patients with complex structural heart disease. The techniques described in this review explore some of the applications, including transseptal puncture for left heart procedures, transcaval for large-bore arterial access from the femoral vein, BASILICA to prevent coronary artery obstruction from TAVR, LAMPOON to prevent LVOT obstruction from TMVR, and ELASTA-Clip to enable TMVR after TEER.

CLINICS CARE POINTS

- Radiofrequency-assisted transseptal access is a simple and safe introduction to transcatheter electrosurgery

- Transcaval access enables large bore arterial access from the femoral vein and has been used for TAVR, TEVAR, and 5.0 Impella insertion

- BASILICA is feasible, safe, and effective at preventing coronary obstruction from TAVR

- LAMPOON prevents LVOT obstruction from TMVR and the appropriate iteration should be considered given the anatomy of each patient
- ELASTA-Clip is a timely novel technique that enables TMVR after TEER

ACKNOWLEDGMENTS

Supported by the National Heart Lung and Blood Institute, National Institutes of Health, USA (Z01-HL006040).

DISCLOSURE

(J.M.Khan), (T.Rogers), and (R.J.Lederman) are co-inventors on patents, assigned to NIH, on catheter devices to lacerate valve leaflets.(A.B.Greenbaum) is a proctor for Edwards Lifesciences, Medtronic, and Abbott Vascular. He has equity in Transmural Systems. (V.C.Babaliaros) is a consultant for Edwards Lifesciences, Abbott Vascular and Transmural Systems, and his employer has research contracts for clinical investigation of transcatheter aortic and mitral devices from Edwards Lifesciences, Abbott Vascular, Medtronic, St Jude Medical, and Boston Scientific. (T.Rogers) is a consultant/proctor for Edwards Lifesciences and Medtronic. He has equity in Transmural Systems. (R.J.Lederman) is the principal investigator on a Cooperative Research and Development Agreement between NIH and Edwards Lifesciences on transcatheter modification of the mitral valve. No other author has a financial conflict of interest related to this research.

REFERENCES

1. Khan JM, Rogers T, Greenbaum AB, et al. Transcatheter electrosurgery: JACC State-of-the-art review. J Am Coll Cardiol 2020;75(12):1455–70.

2. Rosenthal E, Qureshi SA, Chan KC, et al. Radiofrequency-assisted balloon dilatation in patients with pulmonary valve atresia and an intact ventricular septum. Br Heart J 1993;69(4):347–51.

3. Nicholson W, Harvey J, Dhawan R. E-CART (ElectroCautery-assisted re-enTry) of an aorto-ostial right coronary artery chronic total occlusion: first-in-man. JACC Cardiovasc Interv 2016;9(22):2356–8.

4. Khan JM, Rogers T, Eng MH, et al. Guidewire electrosurgery-assisted trans-septal puncture, 2017. Catheter Cardiovasc Interv 2018;91(6):1164–70.

5. Hsu JC, Badhwar N, Gerstenfeld EP, et al. Randomized trial of conventional transseptal needle versus radiofrequency energy needle puncture for left atrial access (the TRAVERSE-LA study). J Am Heart Assoc 2013;2(5):e000428.

6. Carroll JD, Mack MJ, Vemulapalli S, et al. STS-ACC TVT registry of transcatheter aortic valve replacement. J Am Coll Cardiol 2020;76(21):2492–516.

7. Tsilimparis N, Dayama A, Perez S, et al. Iliac conduits for endovascular repair of aortic pathologies. Eur J Vasc Endovasc Surg 2013;45(5):443–8. discussion 9.

8. Lederman RJ, Greenbaum AB, Rogers T, et al. Anatomic suitability for transcaval access based on computed tomography. JACC Cardiovasc Interv 2017;10(1):1–10.

9. Lederman RJ, Babaliaros VC, Greenbaum AB. How to perform transcaval access and closure for transcatheter aortic valve implantation. Catheter Cardiovasc Interv 2015;86(7):1242–54.

10. Greenbaum AB, Babaliaros VC, Chen MY, et al. Transcaval access and closure for transcatheter aortic valve replacement: a prospective investigation. J Am Coll Cardiol 2017;69(5):511–21.

11. Lederman RJ, Babaliaros VC, Rogers T, et al. The fate of transcaval access tracts: 12-month results of the prospective NHLBI transcaval transcatheter aortic valve replacement study. JACC Cardiovasc Interv 2019;12(5):448–56.

12. Fanari Z, Hammami S, Goswami NJ, et al. Percutaneous thoracic aortic aneurysm repair through transcaval aortic access. Catheter Cardiovasc Interv 2017;90(5):806–8.

13. Afana M, Altawil M, Basir M, et al. Transcaval access for the emergency delivery of 5.0 liters per minute mechanical circulatory support in cardiogenic shock. Catheter Cardiovasc Interv 2021;97(3):555–64.

14. Ribeiro HB, Webb JG, Makkar RR, et al. Predictive factors, management, and clinical outcomes of coronary obstruction following transcatheter aortic valve implantation: insights from a large multicenter registry. J Am Coll Cardiol 2013;62(17):1552–62.

15. Khan JM, Dvir D, Greenbaum AB, et al. Transcatheter laceration of aortic leaflets to prevent coronary obstruction during transcatheter aortic valve replacement: concept to first-in-human. JACC Cardiovasc Interv 2018;11(7):677–89.

16. Lederman RJ, Babaliaros VC, Rogers T, et al. Preventing coronary obstruction during transcatheter aortic valve replacement: from computed tomography to BASILICA. JACC Cardiovasc Interv 2019;12(13):1197–216.

17. Khan JM, Greenbaum AB, Babaliaros VC, et al. The BASILICA trial: prospective multicenter investigation of intentional leaflet laceration to prevent TAVR coronary obstruction. JACC Cardiovasc Interv 2019;12(13):1240–52.

18. Khan JM, Greenbaum AB, Babaliaros VC, et al. BASILICA trial: one-year outcomes of transcatheter electrosurgical leaflet laceration to prevent TAVR

coronary obstruction. Circ Cardiovasc Interv 2021; 14(5):e010238.

19. Khan JM, Babaliaros VC, Greenbaum AB, et al. Preventing coronary obstruction during transcatheter aortic valve replacement: results from the multicenter international BASILICA registry. JACC Cardiovasc Interv 2021;14(9):941–8.

20. Khan JM, Bruce CG, Babaliaros VC, et al. TAVR roulette: caution regarding BASILICA laceration for TAVR-in-TAVR. JACC Cardiovasc Interv 2020;13(6): 787–9.

21. Greenbaum AB, Kamioka N, Vavalle JP, et al. Balloon-assisted BASILICA to facilitate redo TAVR. JACC Cardiovasc Interv 2021;14(5):578–80.

22. Kamioka N, Lederman RJ, Khan JM, et al. BI-SILICA during transcatheter aortic valve replacement for noncalcific aortic insufficiency. **JACC Cardiovasc Interv** 2018;11(21):2237–9.

23. Forrestal BJ, Khan JM, Torguson R, et al. Reasons for screen failure for transcatheter mitral valve repair and replacement. Am J Cardiol 2021;148: 130–7.

24. Kohli K, Wei ZA, Sadri V, et al. Dynamic nature of the LVOT following transcatheter mitral valve replacement with LAMPOON: new insights from post-procedure imaging. Eur Heart J Cardiovasc Imaging 2021.

25. Khan JM, Rogers T, Schenke WH, et al. Intentional laceration of the anterior mitral valve leaflet to prevent left ventricular outflow tract obstruction during transcatheter mitral valve replacement: pre-clinical findings. JACC Cardiovasc Interv 2016;9(17):1835–43.

26. Babaliaros VC, Greenbaum AB, Khan JM, et al. Intentional percutaneous laceration of the anterior mitral leaflet to prevent outflow obstruction during transcatheter mitral valve replacement: first-in-human experience. JACC Cardiovasc Interv 2017; 10(8):798–809.

27. Case BC, Lisko JC, Babaliaros VC, et al. LAMPOON techniques to prevent or manage left ventricular outflow tract obstruction in transcatheter mitral valve replacement. Ann Cardiothorac Surg 2021; 10(1):172–9.

28. Lisko JC, Greenbaum AB, Khan JM, et al. Antegrade intentional laceration of the anterior mitral leaflet to prevent left ventricular outflow tract obstruction: a simplified technique from bench to bedside. Circ Cardiovasc Interv 2020;13(6):e008903.

29. Case BC, Khan JM, Satler LF, et al. Tip-to-Base LAMPOON to Prevent left ventricular outflow tract obstruction in valve-in-valve transcatheter mitral valve replacement. JACC Cardiovasc Interv 2020; 13(9):1126–8.

30. Khan JM, Trivedi U, Gomes A, et al. Rescue" LAMPOON to treat transcatheter mitral valve replacement-associated left ventricular outflow tract obstruction. JACC Cardiovasc Interv 2019; 12(13):1283–4.

31. Khan JM, Babaliaros VC, Greenbaum AB, et al. Anterior leaflet laceration to prevent ventricular outflow tract obstruction during transcatheter mitral valve replacement. J Am Coll Cardiol 2019; 73(20):2521–34.

32. Khan JM, Rogers T, Babaliaros VC, et al. Predicting left ventricular outflow tract obstruction despite anterior mitral leaflet resection: the "Skirt Neo-LVOT. JACC Cardiovasc Imaging 2018;11(9):1356–9.

33. Lisko JC, Babaliaros VC, Khan JM, et al. Tip-to-Base LAMPOON for transcatheter mitral valve replacement with a protected mitral annulus. JACC Cardiovasc Interv 2021;14(5):541–50.

34. Khan JM, Lederman RJ, Sanon S, et al. Transcatheter mitral valve replacement after transcatheter electrosurgical laceration of alfieri STItCh (ELASTIC): first-in-human report. JACC Cardiovasc Interv 2018;11(8):808–11.

35. Lisko JC, Greenbaum AB, Guyton RA, et al. electrosurgical detachment of mitraclips from the anterior mitral leaflet prior to transcatheter mitral valve implantation. JACC Cardiovasc Interv 2020;13(20): 2361–70.

Catheter-Based Management of Heart Failure
Pathophysiology and Contemporary Data

Ishan Kamat, MD[a], Alexander G. Hajduczok, MD[b],
Husam Salah, MD[c], Philipp Lurz, MD, PhD[d],
Paul A. Sobotka, MD[e], Marat Fudim, MD[f,g],*

KEYWORDS

- Heart failure - Interventional cardiology - Device therapy - Remote monitoring

---

KEY POINTS

- Device-based therapy for patients with heart failure attempts to address the unmet need whereby pharmacotherapy falls short.
- Implantable remote monitoring devices have shown promise in randomized controlled trials to prevent hospitalizations.
- Interventions include mechanical circulatory support, structural remodeling therapy, diuresis augmentation, and sympathetic modulation.

INTRODUCTION

Pharmacologic advances including quadruple therapy for heart failure (HF) with reduced ejection fraction (HFrEF) reduce mortality and improve clinical outcomes in this population. In patients with HF with preserved ejection fraction (HFpEF), severe HF requires advanced therapies, or acute decompensated HF, pharmacotherapy falls short.[1–4] To address this unmet need, the treatment landscape has favored the development and approval of device-based management.[4] As a result, the application of invasive diagnostic or therapeutic procedures for HF has led to the formation of discipline referred to as interventional HF.[5] We present an overview of recently approved and investigational therapies that will help shape clinical practice in the upcoming years.

REMOTE MONITORING DEVICES

Hemodynamic remote monitoring has emerged to improve rates of hospitalizations for patients with HF. Implantable pulmonary artery (PA) pressure monitoring devices may show a benefit in reducing HF hospitalizations as compared with thoracic impedance-based implantable devices.[6,7] The Chronicle device (Medtronic, Fridley, Minnesota) is an implantable cardiac defibrillator with an additional right ventricular lead used to measure changes in right ventricular pressure that showed improved overall outcomes in meta-analyses of REDUCE-HF and

---

[a] Section of Cardiology, Baylor College of Medicine, 1 Moursund Street, Houston, TX 77030, USA; [b] Department of Cardiology, Thomas Jefferson University Hospital, Philadelphia, PA 19107, USA; [c] Department of Medicine, University of Arkansas for Medical Sciences, 4301 West Markham Street, Little Rock, AR 72205, USA; [d] Department of Cardiology, Heart Center Leipzig, University of Leipzig, Russenstraße 69A, 04289 Leipzig, Germany; [e] Division of Cardiology, Ohio State University, 281 W Lane Avenue, Columbus, OH 43210, USA; [f] Division of Cardiology, Duke University Medical Center, 2301 Erwin Road Durham, NC 27710, USA; [g] Duke Clinical Research Institute, 200 Morris Street, Durham, NC 27701, USA
* Corresponding author. Duke University Medical Center, 2301 Erwin Road Durham, NC 27710.
E-mail address: Marat.fudim@duke.edu

Intervent Cardiol Clin 11 (2022) 267–277
https://doi.org/10.1016/j.iccl.2022.01.005

Abbreviations	
HF	Heart Failure
HFrEF	Heart Failure with reduced ejection fraction
PA	Pulmonary artery
NYHA	New York Heart Association
MR	Mitral regurgitation
LV	Left ventricle
MI	Myocardial infarction
EF	Ejection fraction
GDMT	Guideline-Directed Medical Therapy
PCWP	Pulmonary capillary wedge pressure
IABP	Intra-aortic balloon pump
LVAD	Left ventricular assist device
RVAD	Right ventricular assist device
RDN	Renal denervation
HFpEF	Heart Failure with preserved ejection fraction
CS	Cardiogenic shock
FDA	Food and Drug Administration

COMPASS-HF.[8,9] These studies were not powered to detect mortality benefits, and the ongoing GUIDE-HF trial will hopefully provide more insight into the benefit of PA pressure monitoring in HF.[10] The CHAMPION trial evaluated the efficacy of a wireless implantable PA pressure sensor (Fig. 1, CardioMEMS, Abbott, Chicago, Illinois), demonstrating a reduction in HF hospitalizations (Table 1).[11,12] This device is indicated for monitoring PA pressures heart rate in patients with HF who are exhibiting New York Heart Association (NYHA) Class III symptoms and have been hospitalized in the previous year.[13] Real-world data from the CardioMEMS HF System Post-Approval Study showed that a PA-pressure guided strategy for ambulatory HF management was associated with a lower rate of HF and all-cause hospitalizations with a low number of adverse events across a broad range of patients with symptomatic HF and prior HF hospitalizations.[14]

The Cordella PA Pressure Sensor System (see Fig. 1, Endotronix, Lisle, IL) is an investigational device that is not currently approved for clinical use and uses a similar pressure monitoring strategy to CardioMEMS but differs in that it transmits via a handheld remote rather than having to lay down in bed.[15] The SIRONA trial showed

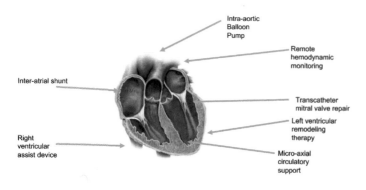

Fig. 1. Intracardiac devices for heart failure management. Remote hemodynamic monitoring devices (Cardio-Mems) measure pulmonary artery pressure to tailor therapy. Transcatheter mitral valve repair (MitraClip), left ventricular remodeling therapy (Revivent TC System), and inter-atrial shunts are solutions for the management of chronic HF. Intra-aortic balloon pumps, right ventricular assist devices (Impella RP, Protek Duo), and micro-axial circulatory support (Impella) can provide circulatory support in cardiogenic shock.

Table 1 Remote monitoring strategies			
Device Category	**Selected Clinical Trials**	**Type**	**Main Outcomes/Conclusions**
CardioMEMS	CHAMPION	RCT	Among patients with recent hospitalization for heart failure, an implantable device to provide daily pulmonary artery hemodynamic information was beneficial in reducing HF hospitalizations (0.44 vs 0.32 per 6 mo).
	GUIDE-HF (ongoing) NCT03387813	RCT	This large RCT will aim to demonstrate the effectiveness of the CardioMEMS™ HF System in an expanded patient population including patients with HF outside of the present indication, but at risk for future HF events or mortality. Goal enrolment: 3600 subjects.
Cordella	SIRONA II (ongoing) NCT04012944	Prospective, single-arm	Aims to establish that the Cordella PA Sensor can be safely delivered, deployed, and remain stable within the pulmonary artery (PA) segment through 30 d postimplant. And will compare Cordella PA Sensor System pressure measurements with standard right heart catheterization (RHC) measurements. Goal enrolment: 60 subjects.

an adequate safety profile of the device and SIRONA II (NCT04012944) will continue to assess device safety and efficacy compared with standardized right heart catheterization measurements (see Table 1).[15]

STRUCTURAL CARDIAC DEVICES/THERAPIES

Transcatheter mitral valve repair

Mitral valve repair for patients with dilated cardiomyopathy and secondary mitral regurgitation (MR) using the MitraClip (see Fig. 1, Abbott, Chicago, IL) has been shown to improve quality of life and decrease morality.[16] In addition to the original FDA indication for primary MR in patients of prohibitive surgical risk, the MitraClip device is now indicated for moderate-to-severe secondary MR due to HF (Table 2).[17] The COAPT trial showed efficacy and met its primary endpoint of HF hospitalizations at 24 months.[18] However, a second randomized controlled trial (MITRA-FR) investigated MitraClip for secondary MR did not show the same clinical outcomes benefit despite being effective at reducing the severity of MR.[19] Differences in trial results could be attributed to subtle differences in inclusion criteria and study design. Overall, patients in COAPT had more severe HF symptoms refractory to medical therapy, less left ventricular (LV) dilatation, and greater degree of MR as compared with patients in MITRA-FR.[18,19] Based on the COAPT results, the FDA approved MitraClip in 2019 for symptomatic

secondary 3+/4+ MR despite optimal medical management for HF.

Left ventricular remodeling therapy

Postmyocardial infarction (MI) remodeling results in pathologic increase LV volume and reduced LV ejection fraction (EF). The Revivent TC System (see Fig. 1, BioVentrix Inc., San Ramon, CA) is an investigative device that provides a novel transcatheter technique to reconstruct the LV by plicating and excluding the fibrous scar to restore LV function. A prospective observational study using this strategy showed a sustained reduction of LV volumes and improvement of LV function, symptoms, and quality of life at 12 months.[20] The REVIVE-HF (NCT03845127) will assess the treatment of ischemic cardiomyopathy induced HF with the Revivent TC System plus Guideline-Directed Medical Therapy (GDMT) compared with GDMT alone (see Table 2).

Interatrial shunt

Interatrial shunts are created between the left and right atria to decompress left atrial pressure (see Fig. 1), a key contributor to worsening symptoms in HF.[21] Currently several devices are in investigational stages (see Table 2). The InterAtrial Shunt Device (IASD, Corvia Medical, Tewksbury, MA) is a nitinol device that is implanted after a standard trans-septal puncture. The REDUCE LAP-HF I trial evaluated IASD safety and feasibility in patients with elevated

Table 2 Structural cardiac devices/therapies			
Device Category	**Selected Clinical Trials**	**Type**	**Main Outcomes/Conclusions**
Mitraclip	COAPT	RCT	Transcatheter mitral valve approximation using the MitraClip on a background of maximally tolerated GDMT was superior to GDMT alone in reducing HF hospitalization and mortality in patients with symptomatic HF with grade 3–4+ MR. Possible reasons for the difference between COAPT and MITRA-FR: patients with COAPT had more severe mitral regurgitation by effective regurgitant orifice area and ventricular dilation.
	MITRA-FR	RCT	Among patients with severe secondary mitral regurgitation, percutaneous mitral regurgitation repair (MitraClip) was not beneficial (no reduction in the composite of death or hospitalization for heart failure).
Revivent TC System	REVIVE-HF (ongoing) NCT03845127	RCT	Ongoing randomized controlled trial (RCT): The purpose of the study is to demonstrate that treatment with the BioVentrix Revivent TC System is more effective than guideline-directed medical therapy for the treatment of ischemic heart failure. Goal enrolment: 180 subjects.
Intra-atrial shunt	REDUCE LAP-HF I	RCT	In patients with heart failure and left ventricular ejection fraction equal to or >40%, a transcatheter interatrial shunt device reduces exercise pulmonary capillary wedge pressure and is safe compared with sham control treatment at 12 mo of follow-up.

pulmonary capillary wedge pressures (PCWP) and at least New York Heart Association (NYHA) class II symptoms.[22] Patients demonstrated improvement in exercise PCWP at 1-month and patency at 1-year and further studies are underway.[22,23]

The V-Wave device (V-Wave Ltd, Caesarea, Israel) is another nitinol-based interatrial shunt system that is similarly delivered after interatrial puncture. Initially, the device included a one-way valve,

but this feature resulted in the loss of patency due to pannus infiltration of the bioprosthetic valve leaflets.[24] The device has been redesigned and initial trialing is underway.

A third device, the atrial flow regulator (AFR, Occlutech, Istanbul, Turkey), is another transseptal leave-behind device that is available in several sizes that have been implemented in several case reports.[25–27] The exact role for timing and size of interatrial shunt will serve as areas of exploration.

ACUTE MECHANICAL CIRCULATORY SUPPORT

Intra-aortic balloon pump

The role of intra-aortic balloon pump (IABP) use has not been clearly defined in RCTs, despite its widespread use in cardiogenic shock (CS) for decades (see Fig. 1). The only large scale randomized study with IABP, the IABP-SHOCK II trial, did not show a clear benefit of IABP use in CS due to acute MI.[28] Thus, the role of IABP to treat acute or chronic HF complicated by CS is unclear. In a retrospective analysis of a single-center using IABP for acute decompensated HF and CS, the 30-day survival in 132 patients was 84.1% (Table 3). This was driven by bridge to LVAD or transplant in 78% of patients with ischemic cardiomyopathy and PA pulsatility index being the most significant predictors of clinical deterioration on IABP.[29] Further RCT-level evidence may help delineate a clear role for IABP in this population, but the overall outcomes given the current landscape are encouraging.

Micro-axial circulatory support

Acute mechanical circulatory support for CS is increasingly used as a bridge to transplant, cardiac function recovery, or long-term left ventricular device implantation. Furthermore, acute percutaneous mechanical support is used as a supportive tool in performing complex, high-risk coronary interventions.[30] The Impella (Abiomed, Danvers, MA) is a micro-axial circulatory support device available in multiple models including the Impella 5.0, and Impella 5.5, and Impella RP (see Fig. 1).[31] These devices are indicated for short term use (14 days) and for CS following acute MI or cardiomyopathy.[32] The Impella 5.0 is introduced through a surgical cutdown through an anastomosed 8 to 10 mm Dacron graft and is placed in the left ventricle in a retrograde fashion through the aortic valve to unload the left ventricle and support mean arterial pressure.[31,33] The impeller pump provides continuous flow from the LV to the ascending aorta through a circulating impeller at a rate of 5.0L/min. The Impella 5.5 can be introduced through the left or right axillary artery and can deliver up to 6.2L/min blood flow. It has no pigtail, reducing the risk of thrombus accumulation or caching chordae tendineae.[30] This allows for longer implantation times.

Often overlooked, RV failure requiring support is common among patients with underlying RV dysfunction and those requiring durable left ventricular assist device (LVAD) support are particularly prone to RV failure (see Table 3).[34] Another Impella model, the Impella RP, is introduced trans-venously to provide right ventricular support and has been used in parallel with left-sided models for biventricular support.[31]

Protek Duo

The Protek Duo (TandemLife, Pittsburgh, PA, USA) is another percutaneous device that serves as a percutaneous right ventricular assist device (RVAD) (see Fig. 1). In a retrospective analysis of Protek Duo use for RV failure at two centers in 17 patients, 23% were weaned from the device, whereas 35% required escalation to a durable RVAD and 41% died. In 12 of the 17 patients, the Protek Duo device was inserted post-LVAD.[35] In a retrospective analysis of Protek Duo use specifically post-LVAD, there was an 81% survival at 1-year and weaning occurred in

Table 3			
Acute mechanical support			
Device Category	**Selected Clinical Trials**	**Type**	**Main Outcomes/Conclusions**
Impella	RELIEF I	Prospective, single-arm	Primary objective was to assess the safety and feasibility of IMPELLA 2.5 in Acute Decompensated Heart Failure patients. Study terminated due to low enrolment.
IABP	Fried et al., 2018. JHLT.	Retrospective	Single-center retrospective study of IABP for acute decompensated HF and CS showed a 30-d survival in 132 patients of 84.1%.
Protek duo	Ravichandran et al., 2018. ASAIO.	Retrospective	In a retrospective analysis of 17 patients with RV failure at two centers, 23% were weaned from the device, 35% required escalation to a durable RVAD, with a mortality rate of 41%.

81% of patients with only 11% requiring conversion to durable RVAD (see Table 3).[36] Additional studies comparing Protek Duo use in acute RV failure, both in the presence and absence of LVAD implantation, are necessary to confirm the efficacy of the device. In addition, head-to-head studies versus durable RVADs would help determine the best acute management strategy for patients with acute RV failure and CS.

CARDIORENAL SYNDROME

Worsening renal function is a complicating factor in HF.[37] Patients with changes in renal function during HF decompensation portends poor outcomes.[37] Thus, improvement in renal perfusion to improve diuresis has become a target for device therapy. Three ways to theoretically improve renal function are through increasing arterial pressure, decreasing venous pressure, or applying negative pressure to the urinary collecting system.[38–40] There are 3 mechanisms of device therapy to manage cardiorenal syndrome: intra-aortic axial flow pump, venous axial flow pump, and ureteral suction collection.

One device aimed at specifically treating worsening renal failure in chronic HF is a 6 mm intra-aortic axial flow pump (Aortix, Procyrion, Houston, Texas). This device is percutaneously implanted in the descending aorta, whereby nitinol anchors affix the pump to the supra-renal aortic wall (Fig. 2).[41] The device is connected to an external motor, supporting up to 5.0 L/min of flow.[42] Because the device entrains an increased pressure gradient across the pump, kidneys experience increased perfusion pressure, leading to increased urinary output. An early small-scale human trial in patients with left ventricular dysfunction undergoing percutaneous coronary intervention demonstrated increased urine production and glomerular filtration rate (Table 4).[38] Further trials to evaluate the efficacy in worsening renal function in HF are underway (NCT04145635).

In contrast to the aortic axial flow pump, the Transcatheter Renal Venous Decongestion system (Magenta Medical, Kadima, Israel) is an axial flow pump placed in renal veins to "pull" fluid worsening renal function in HF (see Fig. 2). In an early small-scale study, the device was temporarily placed in the renal veins of patients with acute decompensated HF and showed improvements in renal blood flow and right atrial pressure. However, changes in urine output varied, so it is unclear whether this device will augment improved diuresis in the face of diuretic resistance (see Table 4).[39]

The third mechanism of augmenting urinary output is applying negative pressure to the urinary collecting system through bilateral ureteral suction catheters (JuxtaFlow, 3ive Labs, Rosewell, GA) in conjunction with diuretic therapy (see Fig. 2). Implementation in an animal model showed increased diuresis, natriuresis, and creatinine clearance (see Table 4).[40]

SYMPATHETIC DENERVATION

Sympathetic overactivation leading to arterial hypertension and increased afterload is thought to be a driving force behind the development of HFpEF.[43,44] Thus, renal denervation (RDN), for which numerous trials have been aimed at treating essential hypertension,[45,46] may be a treatment modality to manage HFpEF (see Fig. 2). Another retrospective study demonstrates that patients had reduced left ventricular mass, improved systolic function, and indices of diastolic function compared with optimal medical therapy after 6 months.[47] In another multicenter study, RDN showed improved in LV circumferential strain.[48] Recently, a retrospective study

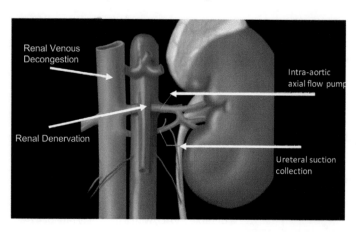

Fig. 2. Extracardiac devices for heart failure management three devices relieve venous congestion, facilitating diuresis. Renal venous decongestion devices (Transcatheter Renal Venous Decongestion System) "pull" blood, intra-aortic axial flow pump (Aortix) would push blood flow, and the ureteral suction collection (JuxtaFlow) is placed in the ureter. Not pictured are splanchnic nerve block and lymphatic drainage.

Table 4
Extracardiac therapies

Device Category	Selected Clinical Trials	Type	Main Outcomes/ Conclusions
Intra-aortic axial flow pump	Aortic CRX Pilot Study (ongoing) NCT04145635	Prospective, single-arm	This prospective, multi-center, nonrandomized feasibility study will evaluate the safety and performance of the Aortix System in patients hospitalized with acute decompensated heart failure and worsening renal function refractory to medical management with persistent congestion. Goal enrolment: 45 subjects.
Transcatheter venous decongestion	TRVD (terminated early) NCT03621436	Prospective, single-arm	Feasibility of the use of a catheter-mounted expandable flow pump to transiently reduce renal venous pressure (for 24 h) in patients with ADHF and reduced LV function. Actual enrollment: 11 subjects.
Lymphatic duct decompression	N/A	Pilot studies (ongoing)	The WhiteSwell system uses a catheter-based system to create a low-pressure region in the thoracic duct to facilitate lymphatic drainage. This may potentiate interstitial decongestion of the lungs, liver, and kidney.
Ureteral suction catheter	VOID-HF (ongoing) NCT04227977	Prospective, single-arm	Feasibility study to evaluate the JuxtaFlow device safety profile and effectiveness in the treatment of hypervolemia associated with ADHF. Goal enrolment: 10 subjects.
Renal Denervation	Kresoja, et al. Circ Heart Failure 2021.	retrospective	Retrospective study on RDN in patients with hypertension with or without HFpEF, demonstrating that RDN led to improvement in N-terminal pro-B-type natriuretic peptide, NYHA class, and myocardial work.

(continued on next page)

Table 4 (continued)			
Device Category	**Selected Clinical Trials**	**Type**	**Main Outcomes/ Conclusions**
Splanchnic Denervation	Splanchnic III (ongoing) NCT04575428 Rebalance-HF (ongoing) NCT04592445	Prospective, single-arm Prospective, Randomized, Sham-controlled	The two studies investigate the safety and feasibility of long-term splanchnic nerve blockade in HFpEF.

analyzed 164 patients with hypertension with or without HFpEF, demonstrating that RDN led to improvement in N-terminal pro-B-type natriuretic peptide, NYHA class, and myocardial work. These benefits seem to be independent of the changes in blood pressure (see Table 4).[49,50] As RDN earns regulatory approval for hypertension management, there may be soon additional trials to evaluate other indications as well.

Splanchnic nerve denervation is leveraging a novel approach to HF treatment. The splanchnic nerve is a branch of the thoracic sympathetic chain that does not directly interact with the heart. Instead, it innervates the abdominal compartment, exhibiting a vasoconstricting effect on the splanchnic vasculature. When inactivated, the abdominal vasculature vasodilates, which serves as a preload reservoir. Early small-scale studies involving temporary nerve block have shown benefits in acute and chronic HF (see Table 4).[51–54]

LYMPHATIC DUCT DECOMPRESSION

Another target for volume removal is the lymphatic duct system.[55] During episodes of decompensated HF, lymphatic drainage is increased to collect interstitial fluid for delivery back to the blood stream.[56] The WhiteSwell device (Galway, Ireland) places a catheter in the thoracic duct connected to an impeller pump to augment lymphatic drainage (see Table 4).[57]

SUMMARY

A variety of nonpharmacologic options are available for the management of acute and chronic HF. As the field expands and more data are generated due to technological advances in device and monitoring, it is possible that catheter-based therapies could become a mainstay of treatment and guidelines in certain clinical scenarios. Some areas, such as CS, may be difficult to study in larger randomized controlled trials with the rapid addition of new devices and therapies. However, if more clinicians are experienced with the use of these therapies and supporting data to guide usage, it may aid in improving overall outcomes for patients. This review serves as an outline for the current options for the management of HF and may pave the way for future innovation.

CLINICS CARE POINTS

- The use of invasive remote hemodynamic monitoring using PA pressure-guided strategies have been shown to reduce all-cause and HF hospitalizations.
- Catheter-guided mitral valve repair for dilated cardiomyopathy with secondary MR has been shown to decrease mortality and improve quality of life.
- Additional randomized controlled trials will help determine the efficacy of multiple device-based strategies for the management of cardiogenic shock

DISCLOSURE

Dr Lurz has received research grants from Edwards Lifesciences, ReCor, and Occlutech. Dr Fudim was supported by the National Heart, Lung, and Blood Institute (NHLBI) (K23HL151744), the American Heart Association (20IPA35310955), Mario Family Award, Duke Chair's Award, Translating Duke Health Award, Bayer, Bodyport, BTG Specialty Pharmaceuticals and Verily. He receives consulting fees from Abbott, Alleviant, Audicor, AxonTherapies, Bayer, Bodyguide, Bodyport, Boston Scientific, CVRx, Daxor, Deerfield Catalyst, Edwards LifeSciences, Feldschuh Foundation, Fire1, Gradient, Intershunt, NXT Biomedical, Pharmacosmos, PreHealth, Shifamed, Splendo, Vironix, Viscardia, Zoll. All other authors have no relevant disclsoures.

REFERENCES

1. Mitter SS, Pinney SP. Advances in the management of acute decompensated heart failure. Med Clin North Am 2020;104:601–14.

2. Tomasoni D, Adamo M, Lombardi CM, et al. Highlights in heart failure. ESC Heart Fail 2019;6:1105–27.

3. Vieira JL, Ventura HO, Mehra MR. Mechanical circulatory support devices in advanced heart failure: 2020 and beyond. Prog Cardiovasc Dis 2020;63:630–9.

4. Zeitler EP, Abraham WT. Novel Devices in Heart Failure: BAT, Atrial Shunts, and Phrenic Nerve Stimulation. JACC Heart Fail 2020;8:251–64.

5. Ahmad U, Lilly SM. Interventional heart failure and hemodynamic monitoring. Heart Fail Clin 2018;14:625–34.

6. Ali O, Hajduczok AG, Boehmer JP. Remote physiologic monitoring for heart failure. Curr Cardiol Rep 2020;22:68.

7. Alotaibi S, Hernandez-Montfort J, Ali OE, et al. Remote monitoring of implantable cardiac devices in heart failure patients: a systematic review and meta-analysis of randomized controlled trials. Heart Fail Rev 2020;25:469–79.

8. Adamson PB, Gold MR, Bennett T, et al. Continuous hemodynamic monitoring in patients with mild to moderate heart failure: results of the reducing decompensation events utilizing intracardiac pressures in patients with chronic heart failure (REDUCEhf) trial. Congest Heart Fail 2011;17:248–54.

9. Bourge RC, Abraham WT, Adamson PB, et al. Randomized controlled trial of an implantable continuous hemodynamic monitor in patients with advanced heart failure: the COMPASS-HF study. J Am Coll Cardiol 2008;51:1073–9.

10. Lindenfeld J, Abraham WT, Maisel A, et al. Hemodynamic-GUIDEd management of Heart Failure (GUIDE-HF). Am Heart J 2019;214:18–27.

11. Abraham WT, Adamson PB, Bourge RC, et al. Wireless pulmonary artery haemodynamic monitoring in chronic heart failure: a randomised controlled trial. Lancet 2011;377:658–66.

12. Abraham WT, Stevenson LW, Bourge RC, et al. Sustained efficacy of pulmonary artery pressure to guide adjustment of chronic heart failure therapy: complete follow-up results from the CHAMPION randomised trial. Lancet 2016;387:453–61.

13. Cowart T. Premarket Approval (PMA): CARDIOMEMS HF PRESSURE MEASUREMENT SYSTEM. 2014. Available at: https://www.accessdata.fda.gov/scripts/cdrh/cfdocs/cfpma/pma.cfm?id=P100045. Accessed August 3, 2021.

14. Shavelle DM, Desai AS, Abraham WT, et al. Lower rates of heart failure and all-cause hospitalizations during pulmonary artery pressure-guided therapy for ambulatory heart failure: One-year outcomes from the CardioMEMS post-approval study. Circ Heart Fail 2020;13:e006863.

15. Mullens W, Sharif F, Dupont M, et al. Digital health care solution for proactive heart failure management with the Cordella Heart Failure System: results of the SIRONA first-in-human study. Eur J Heart Fail 2020;22:1912–9.

16. Boudoulas KD, Vallakati A, Pitsis AA, et al. The use of MitraClip in secondary mitral regurgitation and heart failure. Cardiovasc Revasc Med 2020;21:1606–12.

17. Office of the Commissioner. FDA approves new indication for valve repair device to treat certain heart failure patients with mitral regurgitation. 2019. Available at: https://www.fda.gov/news-events/press-announcements/fda-approves-new-indication-valve-repair-device-treat-certain-heart-failure-patients-mitral. Accessed August 3, 2021.

18. Stone GW, Lindenfeld J, Abraham WT, et al. Transcatheter Mitral-Valve Repair in Patients with Heart Failure. N Engl J Med 2018;379:2307–18.

19. Obadia J-F, Messika-Zeitoun D, Leurent G, et al. Percutaneous repair or medical treatment for secondary mitral regurgitation. N Engl J Med 2018;379:2297–306.

20. Klein P, Anker SD, Wechsler A, et al. Less invasive ventricular reconstruction for ischaemic heart failure. Eur J Heart Fail 2019;21:1638–50.

21. Freed BH, Shah SJ. Stepping out of the left ventricle's shadow: Time to focus on the left atrium in heart failure with preserved ejection fraction. Circ Cardiovasc Imaging 2017;10. https://doi.org/10.1161/CIRCIMAGING.117.006267. Available at:.

22. Feldman T, Mauri L, Kahwash R, et al. Transcatheter interatrial shunt device for the treatment of heart failure with preserved ejection fraction (REDUCE LAP-HF I [Reduce Elevated Left Atrial Pressure in Patients With Heart Failure]): A phase 2, randomized, sham-controlled trial. Circulation 2018;137:364–75.

23. Shah SJ, Feldman T, Ricciardi MJ, et al. One-year safety and clinical outcomes of a transcatheter interatrial shunt device for the treatment of heart failure with preserved ejection fraction in the reduce elevated left atrial pressure in patients with heart failure (REDUCE LAP-HF I) trial: A randomized clinical trial. JAMA Cardiol 2018;3:968–77.

24. Rodés-Cabau J, Bernier M, Amat-Santos IJ, et al. Interatrial shunting for heart failure: Early and late results from the first-in-human experience with the V-Wave system. JACC Cardiovasc Interv 2018;11:2300–10.

25. Piccinelli E, Castro-Verdes MB, Fraisse A, et al. Implantation of an atrial flow regulator in a child on venoarterial extracorporeal membrane oxygenator as a bridge to heart transplant: a case report. J Card Fail 2021;27:364–7.

26. Sivakumar K, Rohitraj GR, Rajendran M, et al. Study of the effect of Occlutech Atrial Flow Regulator on symptoms, hemodynamics, and echocardiographic parameters in advanced pulmonary arterial hypertension. Pulm Circ 2021;11. 2045894021989966.

27. Vanhie E, VandeKerckhove K, Haas NA, et al. Atrial flow regulator for drug-resistant pulmonary hypertension in a young child. Catheter Cardiovasc Interv 2021;97:E830–4.

28. Thiele H, Zeymer U, Neumann F-J, et al. Intra-aortic balloon counterpulsation in acute myocardial infarction complicated by cardiogenic shock (IABP-SHOCK II): final 12 month results of a randomised, open-label trial. Lancet 2013;382:1638–45.

29. Fried JA, Nair A, Takeda K, et al. Clinical and hemodynamic effects of intra-aortic balloon pump therapy in chronic heart failure patients with cardiogenic shock. J Heart Lung Transpl 2018;37:1313–21.

30. Ramzy D, Soltesz E, Anderson M. New surgical circulatory support system outcomes. ASAIO J 2020;66:746–52.

31. Schwartz B, Jain P, Salama M, et al. The rise of endovascular mechanical circulatory support use for cardiogenic shock and high risk coronary intervention: considerations and challenges. Expert Rev Cardiovasc Ther 2021;19:151–64.

32. Bolt W. Premarket approval (PMA): impella 5.5 with smartassist. 2019. Available at: https://www.accessdata.fda.gov/scripts/cdrh/cfdocs/cfpma/pma.cfm?ID=438721. Accessed August 3, 2021.

33. Dudzinsk JE, Gnall E, Kowey PR. A Review of percutaneous mechanical support devices and strategies. Rev Cardiovasc Med 2018;19:21–6.

34. Kormos RL, Teuteberg JJ, Pagani FD, et al. Right ventricular failure in patients with the HeartMate II continuous-flow left ventricular assist device: incidence, risk factors, and effect on outcomes. J Thorac Cardiovasc Surg 2010;139:1316–24.

35. Ravichandran AK, Baran DA, Stelling K, et al. Outcomes with the tandem Protek Duo dual-lumen percutaneous right ventricular assist device. ASAIO J 2018;64:570–2.

36. Salna M, Garan AR, Kirtane AJ, et al. Novel percutaneous dual-lumen cannula-based right ventricular assist device provides effective support for refractory right ventricular failure after left ventricular assist device implantation. Interact Cardiovasc Thorac Surg 2020;30:499–506.

37. Testani JM, Brisco MA, Turner JM, et al. Loop diuretic efficiency: a metric of diuretic responsiveness with prognostic importance in acute decompensated heart failure. Circ Heart Fail 2014;7:261–70.

38. Vora AN, Schuyler Jones W, DeVore AD, et al. First-in-human experience with Aortix intraaortic pump. Catheter Cardiovasc Interv 2019;93:428–33.

39. Vanderheyden M, Bartunek J, Neskovic AN, et al. TRVD Therapy in Acute HF: proof of concept in animal model and initial clinical experience. J Am Coll Cardiol 2021;77:1481–3.

40. Maulion C, Asher J, Moskow J, et al. Renal negative pressure treatment as a novel therapy for cardio-renal syndrome. J Card Fail 2020;26:S6–7.

41. Annamalai SK, Esposito ML, Reyelt LA, et al. Abdominal positioning of the next-generation intra-aortic fluid entrainment pump (Aortix) improves cardiac output in a swine model of heart failure. Circ Heart Fail 2018;11:e005115.

42. Anouti K, Gray W. The aortix device: support in a tube. Catheter Cardiovasc Interv 2019;93:434–5.

43. Verloop WL, Beeftink MMA, Santema BT, et al. A systematic review concerning the relation between the sympathetic nervous system and heart failure with preserved left ventricular ejection fraction. PLoS One 2015;10:e0117332.

44. Chirinos JA, Segers P, Hughes T, et al. Large-artery stiffness in health and disease: JACC state-of-the-art review. J Am Coll Cardiol 2019;74:1237–63.

45. Kandzari DE, Böhm M, Mahfoud F, et al. Effect of renal denervation on blood pressure in the presence of antihypertensive drugs: 6-month efficacy and safety results from the SPYRAL HTN-ON MED proof-of-concept randomised trial. Lancet 2018;391:2346–55.

46. Böhm M, Kario K, Kandzari DE, et al. Efficacy of catheter-based renal denervation in the absence of antihypertensive medications (SPYRAL HTN-OFF MED Pivotal): a multicentre, randomised, sham-controlled trial. Lancet 2020;395:1444–51.

47. Brandt MC, Mahfoud F, Reda S, et al. Renal sympathetic denervation reduces left ventricular hypertrophy and improves cardiac function in patients with resistant hypertension. J Am Coll Cardiol 2012;59:901–9.

48. Mahfoud F, Urban D, Teller D, et al. Effect of renal denervation on left ventricular mass and function in patients with resistant hypertension: data from a multi-centre cardiovascular magnetic resonance imaging trial. Eur Heart J 2014;35. 2224–31b.

49. Kresoja K-P, Rommel K-P, Fengler K, et al. Renal sympathetic denervation in patients with heart failure with preserved ejection fraction. Circ. Heart Fail 2021;14:e007421.

50. Fudim M, Sobotka PA, Piccini JP, et al. Renal denervation for patients with heart failure: Making a full circle. Circ Heart Fail 2021;14:e008301.

51. Fudim M, Patel MR, Boortz-Marx R, et al. Splanchnic nerve block mediated changes in stressed blood volume in heart failure. JACC Heart Fail 2021;9:293–300.

52. Fudim M, Ganesh A, Green C, et al. Splanchnic nerve block for decompensated chronic heart failure: splanchnic-HF. Eur Heart J 2018;39:4255–6.

53. Fudim M, Jones WS, Boortz-Marx RL, et al. Splanchnic nerve block for acute heart failure. Circulation 2018;138:951–3.

54. Fudim M, Boortz-Marx RL, Ganesh A, et al. Splanchnic nerve block for chronic heart failure. JACC Heart Fail 2020;8:742–52.

55. Fudim M, Salah HM, Sathananthan J, et al. Lymphatic dysregulation in patients with heart failure: JACC review topic of the week. J Am Coll Cardiol 2021;78:66–76.

56. Witte MH, Dumont AE, Clauss RH, et al. Lymph circulation in congestive heart failure: effect of external thoracic duct drainage. Circulation 1969;39:723–33.

57. Rosenblum H, Kapur NK, Abraham WT, et al. Conceptual considerations for device-based therapy in acute decompensated heart failure: DRI2P2S. Circ. Heart Fail 2020;13:e006731.

Contemporary Management of Refractory Angina

Rebekah Lantz, DO[a], Odayme Quesada, MD[b], Georgia Mattingly, BA[a], Timothy D. Henry, MD[c],*

KEYWORDS

- Angina • Coronary artery disease • Microvascular

KEY POINTS

- There are 4 main phenotypes of refractory angina (RA): microvascular angina with minimal coronary artery disease (CAD), limited territory at risk, diffuse threadlike CAD, and end-stage CAD.
- Mortality rate in RA is similar to patients with stable angina and therapies should focus on the quality of life.
- Therapies range from pharmacologic to many investigational noninvasive and invasive therapies on the horizon that include, but are not limited to coronary sinus (CS) reduction and cellular therapy.
- Multidisciplinary approach to treatment in specialized clinics that combine expertise from primary and interventional cardiology, cardiovascular imaging, cardiothoracic surgery, and cardiac rehabilitation can improve outcomes in RA.

INTRODUCTION

Refractory angina (RA) is a challenging clinical syndrome. A lack of consistent terminology and specific coding makes it difficult to accurately describe the epidemiology and natural history.[1–4] The ESC Joint Study Group on Treatment of Refractory Angina (RA) defines RA as angina lasting more than 3 months caused by ischemia in patients with coronary artery disease (CAD) not amenable to medical therapy, angioplasty, or coronary artery bypass graft (CABG).[1,2] Others have taken a broader view of RA to include patients with angina due to ischemia with no obstructive CAD (INOCA).[5–8]

With improved recognition and treatment, short and long-term mortality have improved[9] but both quality of life and health care utilization continue to be a challenge and therefore are the major focus of treatment strategies. As the population ages and the number of patients with RA continue to grow, there has been renewed interest in the development of novel treatment strategies.[2–4] We will review the unique phenotypes that constitute RA, discuss the natural history and review the contemporary management strategies currently available and under investigation.

REFRACTORY ANGINA PHENOTYPES

A classification scheme based on specific CAD features has been proposed to allow for a more comprehensive definition of RA.[5] In brief, Phenotype A is microvascular angina with

---

Funding: This work was supported by the National Heart, Lung, and Blood Institute at the National Institutes of Health under award number K23HL151867 (O. Quesada). This content is solely the responsibility of the authors and does not necessarily represent the official views of the National Institutes of Health.

[a] The Lindner Research Center at the Christ Hospital, 2123 Auburn Avenue, Suite 424, Cincinnati, OH 45219, USA;
[b] Women's Heart Program at The Christ Hospital, 2123 Auburn Avenue, Suite 424, Cincinnati, OH 45219, USA;
[c] The Carl and Edyth Lindner Center for Research and Education, The Christ Hospital, 2123 Auburn Avenue, Suite 424, Cincinnati, OH 45219, USA
* Corresponding author.
E-mail address: Tim.Henry@thechristhospital.com
Twitter: @Odayme (O.Q.); @HenrytTimothy (T.D.H.)

minimal CAD; Phenotype B is limited territory at risk as in a chronic total occlusion (CTO); Phenotype C is diffuse threadlike CAD and; Phenotype D is end-stage CAD (Fig. 1).

Phenotype A: Microvascular Angina with Minimal Coronary Artery Disease

Phenotype A includes patients experiencing angina despite nonobstructive CAD.[10–13] INOCA is increasingly recognized as a cause of angina with an estimated prevalence of 3 to 4 million.[11] The mechanism of ischemia without obstructive epicardial CAD is the dysfunction of the coronary microvascular beds in 50% to 75% of patients with INOCA.[10–15] Endothelial-independent coronary microvascular dysfunction (CMD) is identified by impaired hyperemic coronary flow reserve (CFR) in response to adenosine, and endothelial-dependent CMD is the failure of the endothelium to increase coronary blood flow in response to acetylcholine.[10–15] In patients with INOCA, CMD is associated with increased risk of all-cause mortality and major adverse cardiovascular events (MACE).[16] Persistent angina is common in INOCA and associated with worse outcomes.

Phenotype B: Limited Territory at Risk

Phenotype B categorizes patients with ischemic burden in a limited territory due to obstructive CAD.[5] Most of these patients have a CTO of a dominant vessel, side branch, or distal coronary stenoses.[17–19] Despite significant advancements in CTO percutaneous coronary intervention (PCI) techniques, 10% to 25% of patients are not adequately revascularized due to a combination of location, vessel size, and morphology such as diffuse disease resulting in ongoing ischemia and angina. Many of these patients are too high risk for CABG. In addition, redo CABG presents technical difficulties and results in increased perioperative and in-hospital mortality.[20]

Phenotype C: Diffuse Threadlike Coronary Artery Disease

Phenotype C includes patients with diffuse thread-like disease that frequently involves the distal vessels or side branches.[5] This is typical of the long-standing diabetic patients.[21–23] Cardiac transplant vasculopathy is a variant of this phenotype linked to poor clinical outcomes.[24,25] Revascularization options are limited given the diffuse nature of disease, smaller coronary artery diameter, and extensive atherosclerotic disease, resulting in increased adverse outcomes after CABG. The "distal coronary diffuseness score" was proposed by Graham and colleagues[26] to assess the extent of disease, whereby higher scores correlate with lower adjusted survival in the 2 years following CABG.

Phenotype D: End-Stage Coronary Artery Disease

Phenotype D includes patients with advanced CAD typically following multiple revascularization procedures.[5] These patients usually have a history of prior CABG as well as PCI (frequently multiple) with extensive and progressive atherosclerosis. It is also common for patients in this group to be sustained by a single conduit. Male gender, diabetes, and chronic renal failure are risk factors in these patients with significant coronary lesions deemed unsuitable for revascularization based on a study from Olmsted County, Minnesota.[27]

PATHOPHYSIOLOGY OF ANGINA

It is important to understand the pathophysiology of angina for the classification and management of RA. It is well understood that angina develops from an oxygen supply-demand mismatch that activates receptor signals to the brain. Cardiac myocytes respond to this issue of supply-demand by increasing the ischemic threshold by way of adaptive metabolic responses so that ischemia is averted even when hypoperfusion is present. As myocytes experience metabolic demand, healthy cells switch to consume as well as produce metabolic substrates with higher energetic efficiency.[28,29] Meanwhile in compromised cells, this adaptability of coronary myocytes is flawed.[3] In addition, a complex heart-to-brain generation of triggers, elaboration, and final perception of afferent signals from the heart seems to be present. Each component of sensory trigger, cell recognition, and communication component carry a particular role in the subjective anginal experience.[3]

NATURAL HISTORY OF REFRACTORY ANGINA

There are limited data regarding the natural history of RA and predictors of adverse outcomes.[2,4,30–32] It is estimated that 3% to 5% of the US population have angina. Previous studies suggest that 6% to 14% of patients undergoing cardiac catheterization have angina or ischemia that is not amenable to revascularization.[30–32] The no-option patient may be considered so based on a CTO, diffuse CAD, poor distal targets, diffuse vein graft disease, no conduit for bypass, collateral-dependent circulation,

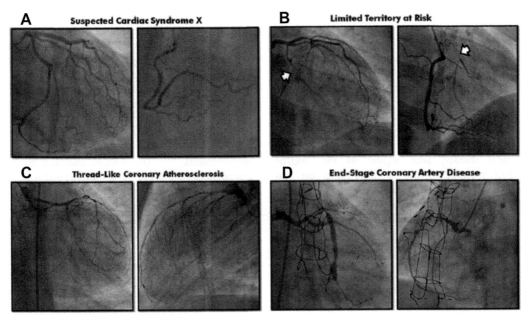

Fig. 1. (A) Microvascular angina with minimal CAD; Phenotype that reflects objective evidence of myocardial ischemia without significant coronary stenosis. (B) Limited territory at risk; Significant stenosis to cause angina but not amenable to PCI and not sufficiently severe to justify first/redo CABG. (C) Diffuse threadlike CAD; less than 1 mm distal runoffs of threadlike appearance from proximal to distal beds. (D) End-stage CAD; Coronaropenia combines proximal stenosis and diffuse atherosclerosis of distal beds. Generally seen in prior, degenerated CABG. (Borrowed with permissions from Jolicoeur EM, Cartier R, Henry TD, et al. Patients With Coronary Artery Disease Unsuitable for Revascularization: Definition, General Principles, and a Classification. Can J Cardiol 2012;29(2 Suppl):S50-S59. Note that Phenotype A is now termed "Microvascular angina with minimal CAD.")

multiple restenosis, and/or comorbidities. A smaller, more specific subpopulation has recently been described as "no-option refractory angina" or NORDA.[33] They typically have disabling class III–IV angina and are without viable options for revascularization. These are the patients that have typically been enrolled in RA clinical trials and represent a more defined population estimated to be 26 to 52,000 in the US.[33] The true prevalence is difficult to know as there is no systematic coding for RA. Therefore, most of the data are derived from single-center registries or extrapolated from "multivessel CAD" or "advanced CAD" reports.

Another important issue is regarding the when and how of categorizing patients as "no-option" for revascularization. CAD is a progressive disease. A recent study from a dedicated RA clinic reported that greater than 20% of "no-option" patients had subsequent revascularization within a median of 2.2 years receiving the diagnosis.[34] New lesions were reported in 48% and new restenosis in 21% of patients. The outcome of patients with new lesions that underwent revascularization was better than for patients with lesions previously felt to be unsuitable for revascularization.[34]

Finally, the long-term outcome for patients with RA was previously considered poor with mortality of 17% at 1-year and 37% at 5-years in 2 registries.[35,36] A more recent article from the Minneapolis Heart Institute RA Registry with more than 1200 patients, reported 17% mortality at 5 years with an annual mortality of 3% to 4% depending on multiple factors including the severity of angina, LVEF and age.[9] Therefore, the contemporary outcome for patients with RA is not much worse than patients with stable angina. Thus, the focus of therapy should include a focus on the quality of life.

MANAGEMENT OF REFRACTORY ANGINA

Treatment modalities vary around the world with available resources and technology. A number of unique treatment options are being investigated around the world.[2–4] (Tables 1 and 2)

Medical Therapies

Regardless of intervention, aggressive risk factor modification is essential including smoking cessation and optimal control of lipids, blood pressure, and diabetes mellitus.[2–4] Guideline-directed antianginal medical therapy should be optimized with beta-blockers (BB), dihydropyridine calcium channel blockers (CCB), and long-acting nitrates. Traditional antianginal medications exert their effects through the reduction of heart rate, blood pressure, and myocardial contractility. Statins may slow the progression of atherosclerosis disease and may also have antianginal effects.[37] Most of the patients with RA have significant CAD and benefit from antiplatelet therapy with aspirin 81 mg and/or P2Y12 platelet inhibitors depending on the timing of previous revascularization and acute coronary syndrome events. The choice of treatment needs to be individualized depending on patients including their underlying risk factors, baseline blood pressure, heart rate, and previous cardiac history.

BB mediate oxygen supply-demand as well as regulate adrenaline's vasodilatory effect. BB block the sympathetic effects of epinephrine and renin release and influence chronotropy, inotropy, dromotropy, and lusitropy. This leads to a decrease in heart rate, contractility, conduction velocity, and relaxation rate. In patients unsuitable for revascularization with previous MI, BB are favored given the associated reduction in postmyocardial infarction mortality.[2,4] CCB block calcium from entering the cardiomyocytes at phase 4, flattening the slope, and effectively decreasing the rate of spontaneous depolarization of cardiac myocytes and the rate of pacemaker firing. CCB also decrease the slope of phase 0, which slows conduction velocity from the atrioventricular node. Note that selective, nondihydropyridine CCB have been associated with increased mortality in patients with low EF. Nitrates specifically cause vasodilation and long-acting nitrates are used for symptom relief in patients with stable angina, while short-acting nitrates are the therapy for choice for acute anginal episodes.

Depending on the country, the availability varies for newer antianginal agents including ivabradine, nicorandil, ranolazine, and trimetazidine. Ivabradine acts on the funny sodium channel and regulates intrinsic chronotropic characteristics of the sinoatrial node.[38,39] It is noninferior to BB in reducing the number of anginal attacks in patients with chronic stable angina; however, it does not reduce blood pressure to the effect that BB do, nor does it exert negative bathmotropic or dromotropic effects. Its superiority to placebo is shown in the ASSOCIATE and BEAUTIFUL trials.[38,39] Nicorandil (not available in the US) is a nicotinamide ester comprising nitrate-like moiety which vasodilates the coronary arteries by the release of nitric oxide (NO) free radicals. It is cardioprotective and promotes the opening of mitochondrial ATP-sensitive potassium channels. Namely, it mimics ischemic preconditioning which is particularly appealing as a substitute for long-acting nitrates.[40] Ranolazine inhibits the late inward sodium current in heart muscle and leads to reductions in intracellular calcium levels, effectively reducing heart wall tension and reducing muscular oxygen requirements.[41,42] The ERICA trial led to the approval of ranolazine by demonstrating a significant reduction in angina and nitroglycerin consumption compared with placebo in patients on maximal doses of amlodipine.[42] It is interesting to note that ranolazine was not initially tested for RA, but a postapproval Ranolazine Refractory Angina Registry suggested effectiveness in the RA population at 3 years.[43] Trimetazidine demonstrated a significant improvement in exercise tolerance and angina compared with placebo in the Trimpol II trial.[44]

Other pharmacologic agents that may show benefit in patients with RA include allopurinol which may lower the risk of ischemic heart disease via an effect on reactive oxygen species and endothelial function.[45] Perhexiline, L-arginine, and testosterone have also been used but there is limited evidence in RA.[2,4] Opiates, while treating sensory pain should generally be avoided given their addiction potential and increased cardiovascular risk with long-term use.[46] Further, the role of depression, anxiety, anticipation, belief, empathy, and pain perception should be accounted for during therapy. Selective serotonin reuptake inhibitors (SSRI) can be used to manage depression and anxiety and have also been hypothesized to prevent microcirculatory dysfunction triggered by inappropriate response to central nervous system stress and the hypothalamus–pituitary–adrenal, though the formal mechanism remains unclear. Tricyclic antidepressants (TCA) and monoamine oxidase inhibitors (MAOi) have been discouraged, however, due to increased QT and arrhythmia potential.[47–49]

Noninvasive Therapies

Beyond medication optimization, there are noninvasive therapies available including enhanced external counter-pulsation (EECP) and low-energy extracorporeal shockwave therapy (ECWT) (Fig. 2).

Enhanced external counter-pulsation

In EECP, coronary blood flow is increased externally with 3 sets of pneumatic cuffs around the

Table 1			
Current treatment modalities in refractory angina			
Current Treatments			
Drug/Therapy Class	**Drug/Therapy Studied**	**Mechanism of Action**	**Phenotypes**
Medical	Beta-blockers	Block sympathetic effects of epinephrine and renin release and influence chronotropy, inotropy, dromotropy, and lusitropy. Decrease heart rate, contractility, conduction velocity, and relaxation rate.	A-D
	Calcium-channel blockers	Block calcium from entering cardiomyocytes at phase 4, flattening slope, and decreasing rate of spontaneous depolarization and pacemaker firing. Decrease the slope of phase 0, which slows conduction velocity from the atrioventricular node.	A-D, step-up therapy
	Nitrates	Vasodilation via nitric oxide free radical pathway, improving oxygen supply to myocardium. Inhibits platelet aggregation.	A-D, step-up therapy
	ACEI & ARB	Acts via the renin–angiotensin–aldosterone system (RAAS) pathway and to reduce small vessel remodeling.	A-D
	Statins	Slow progression of atherosclerotic disease and have antianginal and anti-inflammatory properties.	A-D
	Ivabradine	Acts on the funny sodium channel and regulates intrinsic chronotropic characteristics of the SA node.	A-D, step-up therapy
	Nicorandil	Nicotinamide ester comprising nitrate-like moiety which vasodilates the coronary arteries by the release of nitric oxide free radicals. It is cardioprotective and promotes the opening of mitochondrial ATP-sensitive potassium channels.	A-D, step-up therapy
	Ranolazine	Inhibits late inward sodium current in heart muscle and leads to a reduction in intracellular calcium, reducing heart wall tension and muscular oxygen requirements.	A-D, step-up therapy

(continued on next page)

Table 1 (continued)			
Current Treatments			
Drug/Therapy Class	**Drug/Therapy Studied**	**Mechanism of Action**	**Phenotypes**
Noninvasive	EECP	Coronary blood flow is increased externally with 3 sets of pneumatic cuffs around the lower extremities with counter-pulsation in the diastolic phase as timed air pressure to the lower legs, thighs, and upper thighs sequentially. Increases levels of circulating CD34+ stem cells and endothelial vasoactive factors including NO, VEGF, and FGF-2.	A-D
	ECWT	External application of high amplitude acoustic pressure pulses exerting focal mechanical stress to stimulate angiogenesis and improve ischemia. Uses naturally occurring microbubbles oscillating into and out of cells and collapse in response to acoustics. The stress wave with cavitation effect induces local shear stress which in effect promotes in situ expression of the chemoattractants stromal cell-derived factor 1, VEGF, and NO.	B-D
Invasive	CTO PCI	Creates wider intraluminal area in arteries to restore blood flow and therefore oxygenation to tissues.	B and D

lower extremities. These pneumatic cuffs inflate during diastole to augment coronary flow and deflate in systole to decrease afterload and increase venous return.[50] It is postulated that EECP increases levels of circulating CD34+ stem cells as well as increases a number of vasoactive factors including NO, vascular endothelial growth factor (VEGF), and fibroblast growth factor (FGF-2).[50] An overall improvement in blood pressure has been demonstrated, which may play a role in clinical improvement.[51] Metabolic benefits associated with EECP therapy includes glycemic control with an absolute 1% drop in hemoglobin A1c during the treatment phase that was maintained for up to 6 months in patients with acquired type 2 diabetes mellitus.[52]

The MUST-EECP trial was a randomized sham-controlled trial that led to the approval of EECP in the US for patients with class III–IV angina.[53] Severe angina was shown to be reduced from 89% to 25% with an improvement in the Canadian Cardiovascular Society angina score (CCS).[53] EECP therapy reduced the need for hospitalization by 24% in 1 year and may yield cost savings of about $17,074 after a 35 1-h sessions over 7 weeks. While peripheral vascular disease is a relative contradiction, studies have shown it may be effective for reducing angina with a superimposed peripheral training effect.[50] In summary, EECP results in sustained beneficial effects for reducing angina and improving quality of life.[50–54]

Table 2
Novel treatment modalities in refractory angina

Drug/Therapy Class	Drug/Therapy Studied	Novel Treatments	
		Mechanism of Action	**Phenotypes**
Invasive	Protein & Genetic Approach	Genes altered via viral means for transfer of angiogenetic factors VEGF and FGF.	A-D, Experimental
	Cell Therapy	Autologous CD 34+ bone marrow stem cells are injected directly into ischemic myocardium with in vivo angiogenetic properties.	A-D, Experimental
	TMLR	Surgical, open chest or robotic, laser ablation to create 20–40 transmural channels of 1 mm size in ischemic regions of the myocardium to restore myocardial perfusion.	C-D, Cautious use
	Coronary Sinus Reduction	Direct surgical narrowing of coronary sinus to control restricted drainage of efferent venous blood from the left circulation. Idea to redistribute arterial blood flow to underperfused ischemic myocardium via trans-sinusal pressure gradient.	B-D, Experimental Perhaps A in the future
	Neuromodulation	Chemical, mechanical or electrical means to interrupt a pain signal anywhere in the transmission pathway from the periphery to the brain to alter unfavorable sympathetic afference responsible for vasoconstriction that contributes to ischemia. Includes transcutaneous electrical nerve stimulation (TENS), subcutaneous electrical nerve stimulation (SENS), and spinal cord stimulation (SCS).	C-D, Cautious use
	Cardiac sympathectomy	Surgical severing of the left stellate ganglion as a direct method for interrupting the pain signal from periphery to brain.	C-D, Not recommended

Extracorporeal shockwave therapy/ extracorporeal shockwave myocardial revascularization/cardiac shockwave therapy
Extracorporeal shockwave therapy/extracorporeal shockwave myocardial revascularization/ cardiac shockwave therapy (ECWT/ESMR/ CSWT) is a type of low-energy extracorporeal shockwave therapy that uses acoustic energy shockwaves. A generator accompanies a cardiac ultrasound system so that the targeted area of

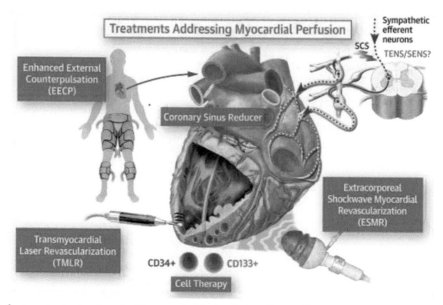

Fig. 2. Refractory angina treatments. (*Borrowed with permissions from* Gallone G, Baldetti L, Tzanis G, et al. Refractory Angina, From Pathophysiology to New Therapeutic Nonpharmacological Technologies. JACC Cardiovasc Interv 2020;13(1):1-19.)

myocardial ischemia can be stimulated.[55] The modality is thought to increase NO production and upregulate vascular mRNA growth factor through focal mechanical stress, in effect stimulating angiogenesis and improving ischemia.[56,57] A single session consists of 1000 shocks, in a sequence of 100 shocks per area. The goal of therapy is for a patient to undergo 9 treatment sessions within 3 months.[55–59] Relative contraindications include bad acoustic windows and left ventricular thrombus. ECWT/ESMR/CSWT has been associated with minimal damage to skin and internal organs with one-tenth the energy of lithotripsy. Overall, the modality seems to be safe and warrants further studies.[3,4]

Minimally Invasive Therapies

These include therapies that target neuromodulatory pathways, and therapeutic angiogenesis whereby the goal is to enhance the body's natural process of neovascularization (see Fig. 2).

Neuromodulation

Neuromodulatory methods use chemical, mechanical or electrical means to interrupt pain signals anywhere in the transmission pathway from the periphery to the brain. The goal is to alter unfavorable sympathetic afferences responsible for vasoconstriction that contributes to symptoms of ischemia. Neuromodulatory methods include transcutaneous electrical nerve

stimulation (TENS), subcutaneous electrical nerve stimulation (SENS), spinal cord stimulation (SCS), and cardiac sympathectomy of the left stellate ganglion.[1–4] Overall results are conflicting, but most of evidence is with SCS which previously received a recommendation from the European Society of Cardiology (ESC).[1]

TENS exploits low-intensity electrical currents by chest electrodes to stimulate large-diameter afferent fibers. In theory, the afferent pain signal is suppressed, and pain is replaced with a vibrating sensation. In return, afterload is reduced by systemic vasodilatation likely due to reduced efferent sympathetic activity. TENS is not definitive therapy and leads to SENS or SCS typically.[3] SENS is a common modality for noncardiac chronic pain disorders. When applied to RA, peripheral subcutaneous multipolar electrodes are implanted parasternally at the location of subjective angina and tunneled to a pulse generator in the upper abdomen. SENS is feasible, effective, and safe; however, evidence is limited to small trials.[3] SCS has been used most frequently for patients with RA. In the small randomized single-blind ESBY trial, 104 patients were randomized to CABG or SCS. SCS had similar quality of life and survival benefit to CABG and may be an effective option for patients at increased surgical risk .[60] Although SCS was previously recommended as a treatment of drive for RA by the ESC, the only randomized, sham-controlled, single-blind trial stopped early due to slow enrollment and showed no significant difference between groups.[61] Lastly, although cardiac sympathectomy of the left cervicothoracic/stellate ganglion has been proposed, there are limited data to support benefit and concerns regarding safety.

Therapeutic angiogenesis

Therapeutic angiogenesis is the use of protein, gene, or cell therapy to enhance the natural process of angiogenesis.[2–4] Theoretically, this is an attractive therapy for RA as the symptoms result from inadequate myocardial perfusion. The initial studies were with proangiogenic growth factors given via intracoronary perfusion nearly 20 years ago, but short half-life was a major limitation.[62,63] This led to a large number of gene therapy trials using both naked DNA plasmid as well as adenovirus vectors delivered intracoronary or by direct intramyocardial injection either via themini-thoracotomy or by percutaneous endomyocardial delivery. The most extensive experience was with an adenovirus encoding FGF-4, the AGENT trials.[64] AGENT III and IV were randomized, placebo-controlled trials with a total of 532 patients treated with IC delivery of Ad5 FGF-4 versus placebo. While overall the primary endpoint, total exercise duration, was not significantly improved, there was a significant improvement in angina at 1 year in both dose groups and a significant improvement in exercise time in women.[65] Another gene therapy trial of note, is the REVASC trial which demonstrated an improvement in time to exercise time (0.8 minute increase vs −0.1 in controls) in patients treated with an adenovirus encoding VEGF121 via mini-thoracotomy with intramyocardial delivery[67]. These results laid the groundwork for the ongoing Xylocor trial (NCT04125732) that is testing an adenovirus vector encoding for multiple isoforms of VEGF.

The gene therapy experience gave way to extensive investigation of cell therapy based on strong preclinical data demonstrating the ability of stem cells to improve myocardial perfusion. The most extensive experience is with the CD34+ cell, an autologous bone marrow-derived mononuclear cell.[2–4,66–70] These cells are mobilized with granulocyte colony-stimulating factor (G-CSF) and collected by leukapheresis. They are then injected either directly into the ischemic myocardium using percutaneous endomyocardial injection d via intracoronary infusion. Three consecutive randomized, double-blinded, placebo-controlled trials in the US demonstrated the safety of intramyocardial delivery of auto-CD34+ cells and significant improvement in short and long-term anginal frequency and total exercise time in patients with obstructive CAD and CCS class III–IV RA.[66–68] A patient-level meta-analysis of the 304 patients randomized in the 3 three trials demonstrated significant improvement in anginal frequency, total exercise time and a reduction in mortality.[69]

CD34+ cell therapy is also currently being investigated for microvascular angina (Phenotype A) based on the preclinical ability of CD34+ cells to repair microvascular in patients with ischemic tissues by promoting vascular repair and angiogenesis.[70,71] A recent 2-center, phase 1 feasibility, and safety trial (ESCAPE-CMD) using autologous CD34+stem cells in patients with INOCA with endothelial-independent CMD demonstrated a significant improvement in CFR (2.08 ± 0.32–2.68 ± 0.79) at 6 months that correlated with improvement in angina and quality of life.[71] CD133+ is another bone-marrow-derived cell therapy has also shown promise with significant improvement in angina symptoms, myocardial perfusion, and PET-CT function in RECARDIO.[72]

Overall multiple metanalyses support the use of cell therapy for patients with RA. Cell therapy is approved in a limited number of countries around the world with variable reimbrusement.[33,69,73]

Invasive Therapies

There are also a number of invasive approaches to the treatment of RA.

Chronic total occlusion percutaneous coronary intervention

There have been considerable advances in the treatment of patients with CTO are present in 60% to 80% of patients with RA. With experienced providers and a catheterization laboratory team, successful recanalization can be achieved in up to 90% of appropriately selected patients.[74–76] Current guidelines recommend CTO PCI for patients unsuitable for CABG who have documented large ischemic burden and remain symptomatic despite optimal guideline-directed medical therapy. CTO PCI is associated with less residual or recurrent angina at 12 to 36 months, improvement in exercise time at 12 months, and greater treatment satisfaction than patients with failed PCI.[74–76] The DECISION CTO randomized 417 patients to CTO PCI versus 398 patients to no PCI strategy. Nearly 20% of patients crossed over and there was a

91% success rate. Patients in both groups had PCI of non-CTO lesions. At a median 4-year follow-up, there were no differences in MACE (22.3% vs 22.4%) and both groups had improvements in QOL. It is important to note that these were not specifically RA patients.

CTO PCI is not without its complications, including MI, perforation, distal bed embolization, and death. CTO PCI should be considered an integral part of a RA program.

Coronary sinus reduction

Ninety percent of the pressure drop along healthy coronary circulation occurs between the prearterioles and the CS. Importantly, an imbalance in regional capillary pressure and arterial blood flow redistributes underperfused ischemic myocardium via the trans-sinusal pressure gradient.[2–4,77–79] The coronary sinus reducer (CSR) is a balloon-expandable hourglass-shaped stent that is implanted to create an outflow gradient in the CS. This percutaneous approach is based on the original principles of the BECK procedure which was a surgical narrowing of the CS. The Phase 2 double-blind COSIRA trial enrolled 104 patients randomized to the CSR versus a sham-controlled procedure and demonstrated a significant improvement in angina and QOL.[78]

Real-world data across multiple centers confirm the safety and efficacy of the procedure with a success rate of 98%, without severe periprocedural complications. Responders have a 70% to 85% rate of symptomatic improvement at 1 to 2-year follow-up.[77,78]

The device is not approved in the US but has been implanted in greater than 3000 patients worldwide demonstrating excellent safety and clinical improvements in angina similar to the COSIRA trial.[77–79] In 2018, an FDA panel agreed there was evidence for safety but recommended additional efficacy data was needed and therefore the COSIRA-2 trial (NCT05102019), a large sham-controlled trial recently began in the US and Canada.

Transmyocardial laser revascularization (TMR)

TMR involves surgical open chest or percutaneous myocardial laser ablation to create 20 to 40 transmural channels of 1 mm size in ischemic regions of the myocardium to restore myocardial perfusion.[2–4,80,81] The proposed benefit of TMR includes injury-stimulating angiogenesis and/or denervation. Surgical TMR is approved for the treatment of RA based on multiple trials randomized against medical therapy with only one sham-controlled trial.[2–4]

However, in the DIRECT trial, there was no benefit for percutaneous TMR over sham in either angina reduction or exercise time and there was an increase in morbidity.[81] Therefore, enthusiasm for TMR waned.

TMR is contraindicated in patients with low ejection fraction or recent MI because morbidity and mortality are substantially increased. It is also not recommended in Europe, whereas TMR with or without CABG is FDA approved for RA treatment as level IIB recommendation in the ACA/AHA 2012 guideline for stable CAD.[82] It is seldom used alone but occasionally used in conjunction with CABG at this time in the US.

Multidisciplinary team

There is evidence that a multidisciplinary team approach in specialized clinics with trained providers including primary and interventional cardiology, cardiovascular imaging, cardiothoracic surgery, and cardiac rehabilitation may improve clinical outcomes in patients with RA.[4,83,84] Primary care providers also contribute by assuring optimal risk factor modification as well as treatment of depression throughout the process of this chronic and debilitating disease. The ideal treatment of RA includes optimized medical therapy with risk factor modification, antiplatelet, and antianginal therapy in conjunction with state-of-the-art surgical and percutaneous revascularization. Still, a substantial number of patients are left with debilitating symptoms and centers that have a full range of novel therapies under investigation can provide options for the "no-option" patient.

SUMMARY

RA is a heterogenous population with 4 distinct phenotypes: Microvascular angina with minimal CAD (phenotype A), limited territory at-risk/ CTO (phenotype B), diffuse threadlike CAD/ DM (phenotype C), and end-stage CAD (phenotype D). Each phenotype presents a different treatment challenge. As patients survive longer with improved therapies, quality of life becomes an increasingly more important goal for the management of RA. Fortunately, a wide range of novel pharmacologic, noninvasive, and invasive therapies are under investigation. A multidisciplinary team care approach has distinct advantages to care for this challenging patient population. More centers with specialized programs for RA including expertise in complex and novel treatments are needed.

CLINICS CARE POINTS

- Initial steps with the treatment of refactors angina patients include aggressive risk factor modifications, antianginal therapy, and review of revascularization options.
- Although clinical outcomes have improved these patients have severe limitations in their quality of life and high resource utilization with limited treatment options.
- Therefore, specialized clinics with novel clinically available and investigative therapies can provide options for the "no-option patient."

REFERENCES

1. Mannheimer C, Camici P, Chester MR, et al. The problem of chronic refractory angina. Eur Heart J 2002;23:355–70.
2. Henry TD, Satran D, Jolicoeur EM. Treatment of refractory angina in patients not suitable for revascularization. Nat Rev Cardiol 2014;11:78–95.
3. Gallone G, Baldetti L, Tzanis G, et al. Refractory angina, from pathophysiology to new therapeutic nonpharmacological technologies. JACC Cardiovascl Interv 2020;13:1–19.
4. Povsic TJ, Henry TD, Ohman EM. Therapeutic approaches for the no-option refractory angina patient. Circ Cardiovasc Interv 2021;14:e009002.
5. Jolicoeur EM, Cartier R, Henry TD, et al. Patients with coronary artery disease unsuitable for revascularization: definition, general principles, and a classification. Can J Cardiol 2012;29(2 Suppl):S50–9.
6. Corcoran D, Young R, Adlam, et al. Coronary microvascular dysfunction in patients with stable coronary artery disease: the CE-MARC 2 coronary physiology sub-study. Int J Cardiol 2018;266:7–14.
7. Sara JD, Widmer RJ, Matsuzawa Y, et al. Prevalence of coronary microvascular dysfunction among patients with chest pain and nonobstructive coronary artery disease. JACC Cardiovasc Interv 2015;8:1445–53.
8. Murthy VL, Naya M, Taqueti VR, et al. Effects of sex on coronary microvascular dysfunction and cardiac outcomes. Circulation 2014;129:2518–27.
9. Henry TD, Satran D, Hodges JS, et al. Long-term survival in patients with refractory angina. Eur Heart J 2013;34:2683–8.
10. Kunadian V, Chieffo A, Camici PG, et al. An EAPCI Expert Consensus Document on Ischaemia with Non-Obstructive Coronary Arteries in Collaboration with European Society of Cardiology Working Group on Coronary Pathophysiology & Microcirculation Endorsed by Coronary Vasomotor Disorders International. EuroIntervention 2021;16:1049–69.
11. Bairey Merz CN, Pepine CJ, Walsh MN, et al. Ischemia and No Obstructive Coronary Artery Disease (INOCA): developing Evidence-Based Therapies and Research Agenda for the Next Decade. Circulation 2017;135:1075–92.
12. Shaw LJ, Shaw RE, Merz CNB, et al. Impact of ethnicity and gender differences on angiographic coronary artery disease prevalence and in-hospital mortality in the American College of Cardiology-National Cardiovascular Data Registry. Circulation 2008;117:1787–801.
13. Pepine CJ, Anderson RD, Sharaf BL, et al. Coronary microvascular reactivity to adenosine predicts adverse outcome in women evaluated for suspected ischemia results from the National Heart, Lung and Blood Institute WISE (Women's Ischemia Syndrome Evaluation) study. J Am Coll Cardiol 2010;55:2825–32.
14. del Buono MG, Montone RA, Camilli M, et al. Coronary microvascular dysfunction across the spectrum of cardiovascular diseases: JACC State-of-the-art review. J Am Coll Cardiol 2021;78:1352–71.
15. Widmer RJ, Samuels B, Samady H, et al. The functional assessment of patients with non-obstructive coronary artery disease: expert review from an international microcirculation working group. EuroIntervention 2019;14:1694–702.
16. Jespersen L, Hvelplund A, Abildstrom SZ, et al. Stable angina pectoris with no obstructive coronary artery disease is associated with increased risks of major adverse cardiovascular events. Eur Heart J 2012;33:734–44.
17. Campeau L, Lesperance J, Hermann J, et al. Loss of the improvement of angina between 1 and 7 years after aortocoronary bypass surgery: correlations with changes in vein grafts and in coronary arteries. Circulation 1979;60(2 Pt 2):1–5.
18. Brilakis ES, Mashayekhi K, Tsuchikane E, et al. Guiding principles for chronic total occlusion percutaneous coronary intervention: a global expert consensus document. Circulation 2019;140:420–33.
19. Vescovo GM, Zivelonghi C, Scott B, et al. Percutaneous coronary intervention for chronic total occlusion. US Cardiol Rev 2020;14:e11.
20. Mohamed MO, Shoaib A, Gogas B, et al. Trends of repeat revascularization choice in patients with prior coronary artery bypass surgery. Catheter Cardiovasc Interv 2020;98:470–80.
21. Farkouh ME, Domanski M, Dangas GD, et al. Long-term survival following multivessel revascularization in patients with diabetes: the FREEDOM follow-on study. J Am Coll Cardiol 2019;73:629–38.

22. Daemen J, Kuck KH, Macaya C, et al. Multivessel coronary revascularization in patients with and without diabetes mellitus: 3-year follow-up of the ARTS-II (Arterial Revascularization Therapies Study-Part II) trial. J Am Coll Cardiol 2008;52: 1957–67.

23. Kapur A, Hall RJ, Malik IS, et al. Randomized comparison of percutaneous coronary intervention with coronary artery bypass grafting in diabetic patients. 1-year results of the CARDia (Coronary Artery Revascularization in Diabetes) trial. J Am Coll Cardiol 2010;55:432–40.

24. Schmauss D, Weis M. Cardiac Allograft Vasculopathy: Recent Developments. Circulation 2008;117: 2131–41.

25. Shetty M, Chowdhury YS. Heart Transplantation Allograft Vasculopathy, vol. 1. Treasure Island (FL): StatPearls Publishing; 2021.

26. Graham MM, Chambers RJ, Davies RF. Angiographic quantification of diffuse coronary artery disease: reliability and prognostic value for bypass operations. J Thorac Cardiovasc Surg 1999;118:618–27.

27. Kiernan TJ, Boilson BA, Sandhu GS, et al. Nonrevascularizable coronary artery disease following coronary artery bypass graft surgery: a population based study in Olmsted, Minnesota. Coron Artery Dis 2009;20:106–11.

28. Fallovollita JA, Malm BJ, Canty JM. Hibernating myocardium retains metabolic and contractile reserve despite regional reductions in flow, function and oxygen consumption at rest. Circ Res 2003;92:48–55.

29. Standley W. Changes in cardiac metabolism: a critical step from stable angina to ischaemic cardiomyopathy. Eur Heart J Suppl 2001;3(Suppl O):O2–7.

30. Mukherjee D, Bhatt DL, Roe MT, et al. Direct myocardial revascularization and angiogenesis—how many patients might be eligible? Am J Cardiol 1999;84:598–600.

31. Williams B, Menon M, Satran D, et al. Patients with coronary artery disease not amenable to traditional revascularization: Prevalence and 3-year mortality. Catheter Cardiovasc Interv 2010;75:886–91.

32. Lenzen M, op Reimer WS, Norekvål TM, et al. Pharmacological Treatment and Perceived Health Status During 1-Year Follow Up in Patients Diagnosed with Coronary Artery Disease, But Ineligible for Revascularization: Results from the Euro Heart Survey on Coronary Revascularization. Eur J Cardiovasc Nurs 2006;5:115–21.

33. Benck L, Henry TD. CD34+ Cell therapy for no-option refractory disabling angina: time for FDA approval? Cardiovasc Revasc Med 2019;20:177–8.

34. Sharma R, Tradewell M, Kohl LP, et al. Revascularization in "no option" patients with refractory angina: Frequency, etiology and outcomes. Catheter Cardiovasc Interv 2018;92:1215–9.

35. Mukherjee D, Comella K, Bhatt DL, et al. Clinical outcome of a cohort of patients eligible for therapeutic angiogenesis or transmyocardial revascularization. Am Heart J 2001;142:72–4.

36. Cavender MA, Alexander KP, Broderick S, et al. Long-term morbidity and mortality among medically managed patients with angina and multivessel coronary artery disease. Am Heart J 2009;158:933–40.

37. Deanfield JE, Sellier P, Thaulow E, et al. Potent anti-ischaemic effects of statins in chronic stable angina: incremental benefit beyond lipid lowering? Eur Heart J 2010;31:2650–9.

38. Tardif JC, Ponikowski P, Kahan T. Efficacy of the I(f) current inhibitor ivabradine in patient with stable angina receiving beta-blocker therapy: a 4-month, andomized, double-blind, placebo-controlled trial. Eur Heart J 2009;30:540–8.

39. Fox K, Ford I, Steg PG, et al. Ivabradine for patients with stable coronary artery disease and left-ventricular systolic dysfunction (BEAUTIFUL): a randomised, double-blind, placebo-controlled trial. Lancet 2008;372(9641):807–16.

40. IONA Study Group. Trial to show the impact of nicorandil in angina (IONA): design, methodology, and management. Heart 2001;85(6):e9.

41. Chaitman BR, Pepine CJ, Parker JO, et al. Effects of ranolazine with atenolol, amlodipine, or diltiazem on exercise tolerance and angina frequency in patients with severe chronic angina: a randomized controlled trial. JAMA 2004;291:309–16.

42. Stone PH, Gratsiansky NA, Blokhin A, et al. Antianginal efficacy of ranolazine when added to treatment with amlodipine: the ERICA (Efficacy of Ranolazine in Chronic Angina) trial. J Am Coll Cardiol 2006;48:566–75.

43. Storey KM, Wang J, Garberich RF, et al. Long-Term (3 Years) Outcomes of ranolazine therapy for refractory angina pectoris (from the Ranolazine Refractory Registry). Am J Cardiol 2020;129:1–4.

44. Szwed H, Sadowski Z, Elikowski W, et al. Combination treatment in stable effort angina using trimetazidine and metoprolol. Results of a randomized, double-blind, multicentre study (TRIMPOL II). Eur Heart J 2001;22:2267–74.

45. Zdenghea M, Sitar-Taut A, Cismaru G, et al. Xanthine oxidase inhibitors in ischaemic heart disease. Cardiovasc J Afr 2017;28:201–4.

46. Hermann CK, Eriksen J. Opioid treatment of pain in angina pectoris. Ugeskr Laeger 2002;164:2297–8.

47. Celano CM, Huffman JC. Depression and cardiac disease: a review. Cardiol Rev 2011;19:130–42.

48. Practice guideline for the treatment of patients with major depressive disorder. 3rd edition. American Psychiatric Association; 2010.

49. Taylor DM, Paton C, Kapur S. The maudsley prescribing guidelines in psychiatry. 12th Edition. Hoboken: Wiley-Blackwell; 2015.

50. Michaels AD, McCullough PA, Soran OZ, et al. Primer: practical approach to the selection of patients for and application of EECP. Nat Clin Pract Cardiovasc Med 2006;3:623–32.

51. Campbell AR, Satran D, Zenovich AG, et al. Enhanced external counterpulsation improves systolic blood pressure in patients with refractory angina. Am Heart J 2008;156:1217–22.

52. Ahlbom M, Hagerman I, Stahlberg M, et al. Increases in cardiac output and oxygen consumption during enhanced external counterpulsation. Heart Lung Circ 2016;25:1133–6.

53. Arora RR, Chou TM, Jain D, et al. The multicenter study of enhanced external counterpulsation (MUST-EECP): effect of EECP on exercise-induced myocardial ischemia and anginal episodes. J Am Coll Cardiol 1999;33:1833–40.

54. Sinvhal RM, Gowda RM, Khan IA. Enhanced external counterpulsation for refractory angina pectoris. Heart 2003;89:830–3.

55. Alunni G, Marra S, Meynet I, et al. The beneficial effect of extracorporeal shockwave myocardial revascularization in patients with refractory angina. Cardiovasc Revasc Med 2015;16:6–11.

56. Schmid JP, Capoferri M, Wahl A, et al. Cardiac shock wave therapy for chronic refractory angina pectoris. A prospective placebo-controlled randomized trial. Cardiovasc Ther 2013;31:e1–6.

57. Vainer J, Habets JH, Schalla S, et al. Cardiac shockwave therapy in patients with chronic refractory angina pectoris. Neth Heart J 2016;24: 343–9.

58. Kikuchi Y, Ito K, Ito Y, et al. Double-blind and placebo-controlled study of the effectiveness and safety of extracorporeal cardiac shock wave therapy for severe angina pectoris. Circ J 2010;74:589–91.

59. Burneikaite G, Shkolnik E, Celutkiene J, et al. Cardiac shock-wave therapy in the treatment of coronary artery disease: systematic review and meta-analysis. Cardiovasc Ultrasound 2017;15:11.

60. Ekre O, Norrsell TE, Wahrborg P, et al. Long-term effects of spinal cord stimulation and coronary artery bypass grafting on quality of life and survival in the ESBY study. Eur Heart J 2002;23:1938–45.

61. Zipes DP, Svorkdal N, Berman D, et al. Spincal cord stimulation therapy for patients with refractory angina who are not candidates for revascularization. Neuromodulation 2012;15:550–8.

62. Henry TD, Annex BH, McKendall GR, et al. VIVA Investigators. The VIVA trial: vascular endothelial growth factor in ischemia for vascular angiogenesis. Circulation 2003;107:1359–65.

63. Simons M, Annex BH, Laham RJ, et al. Pharmacological treatment of coronary artery disease with recombinant fibroblast growth factor-2: double-blind, randomized, controlled clinical trial. Circulation 2002;105:788–93.

64. Henry TD, Grines CL, Watkins MW, et al. Effects of Ad5FGF-4 in patients with angina: an analysis of pooled data from the AGENT-3 and AGENT-4 trials. J Am Coll Cardiol 2007;50:1038–46.

65. Stewart DJ, Hilton JD, Arnold JM, et al. Angiogenic gene therapy in patients with nonrevascularizable ischemic heart disease: a phase 2 randomized, controlled trial of AdVEGF(121) (AdVEGF121) versus maximum medical treatment. Gene Ther 2006;13:1503–11.

66. Losordo DW, Schatz RA, White CJ, et al. Intramyocardial Transplantation of Autologous CD34+ Stem Cells for Intractable Angina: a Phase I/IIa Double-Blind, Randomized Controlled Trial. Circulation 2007;115:3165–72.

67. Losordo DW, Henry TD, Davidson C, et al. Intramyocardial, Autologous CD34+ Cell therapy for refractory angina. Circ Res 2011;109:428–36.

68. Povsic TJ, Henry TD, Traverse JH, et al. The RENEW Trial: Efficacy and Safety of Intramyocardial Autologous CD34(+) Cell Administration in Patients With Refractory Angina. JACC Cardiovasc Interv 2016;9:1576–85.

69. Henry TD, Losordo DW, Traverse JH, et al. Autologous CD34+ cell therapy improves exercise capacity, angina frequency and reduces mortality in no-option refractory angina: a patient-level pooled analysis of randomized double-blinded trials. Eur Heart J 2018;9:2208–16.

70. Rai B, Shukla J, Henry TD, et al. Angiogenic CD34 Stem Cell Therapy in Coronary Microvascular Repair—A Systematic Review. Cells 2021;10:1137.

71. Henry TD, Bairey Merz CN, Wei J, et al. Autologous CD34+ Stem Cell Therapy Increases Coronary Flow Reserve and Reduces Angina in Patients With Coronary Microvascular Dysfunction. Circ Cardiovasc Interv 2022 Feb;15(2):e010802. https://doi.org/10.1161/CIRCINTERVENTIONS.121.010802. Epub 2022 Jan 23. PMID: 35067072; PMCID: PMC8843403.

72. Bassetti B, Carbucicchio C, Catto V, et al. Linking cell function with perfusion: insights from the transcatheter delivery of bone marrow-derived CD133+ cells in ischemic refractory cardiomyopathy trial (RECARDIO). Stem Cell Res Ther 2018;9:235.

73. Fisher SA, Dorée C, Brunskill SJ, et al. Bone marrow stem cell treatment for ischemic heart disease in patients with no option of revascularization: a systematic review and meta-analysis. PLoS One 2013; 8:e64669.

74. Joyal D, Afilalo J, Rinfret S. Effectiveness of recanalization of chronic total occlusions: a systematic review and meta-analysis. Am Heart J 2010;160: 179–87.

75. Werner GS, Martin-Yuste V, Hildick-Smith D, et al. A randomized multicentre trial to compare revascularization with optimal medical therapy for the

treatment of chronic total coronary occlusions. Eur Heart J 2018;39:2484–93.

76. Lee SW, Lee PH, Ahn JM, et al. Randomized trial evaluating percutaneous coronary intervention for the treatment of chronic total occlusion. Circulation 2019;139:1674–83.

77. Giannini F, Baldetti L, Konigstein M, et al. Safety and efficacy of the reducer: a multi-center clinical registry - REDUCE study. Int J Cardiol 2018;269:40–4.

78. Giannini F, Baldetti L, Ponticelli F, et al. Coronary sinus reducer implantation for the treatment of chronic refractory angina: a single center experience. J Am Coll Cardiol Intv 2018;11:784–92.

79. Verheye S, Jolicoeur EM, Behan MW, et al. Efficacy of a device to narrow the coronary sinus in refractory angina. N Engl J Med 2015;372:519–27.

80. Szatkowski A, Ndubuka-Irobunda C, Oesterle SN, et al. Transmyocardial laser revascularization: a review of basic and clinical aspects. Am J Cardiovasc Drugs 2002;2:255–66.

81. Leon MB, Kornowski R, Downey WE, et al. A blinded, randomized, placebo-controlled trial of percutaneous laser myocardial revascularization to improve angina symptoms in patients with severe coronary disease. J Am Coll Cardiol 2005;46: 1812–9.

82. Fihn SD, Gardin JM, Abrams J, et al. 2012 ACCF/AHA/ACP/AATS/PCNA/SCAI/STS Guideline for the Diagnosis and Management of Patients With Stable Ischemic Heart Disease: Executive Summary: a report of the American College of Cardiology Foundation/American Heart Association Task Force of Practice Guidelines, and the American College of Physicians, American Association for Thoracic Surgery, Preventive Cardiovascular Nurses Association, Society for Cardiovascular Angiography and Interventions, and Society of Thoracic Surgeons. J Am Coll Cardiol 2012;60:2564–603.

83. Bennett NM, Rutten-Ramos S, Arndt TL, et al. Health status and quality of life of patients enrolled in a specialized refractory angina clinic. J Minneapolis Heart Inst Found 2019;2:4–8.

84. Riley RF, Kereiakes DJ, Henry TD. More data than options for the "no-option" refractory angina patient in the United States. Circ Res 2019;124:1689–91.

Percutaneous Treatments for Pulmonary Hypertension

Reviewing the Growing Procedural Role for Interventional Cardiology

S. Nabeel Hyder, MD[a], Saurav Chatterjee, MD[b],
Vikas Aggarwal, MD, MPH[a],*

KEYWORDS

- Review • Pulmonary hypertension • Chronic thromboembolic disease • Pulmonary denervation
- Balloon pulmonary angioplasty • Atrial septostomy • Interventional cardiology
- Percutaneous therapy

KEY POINTS

- Balloon pulmonary angioplasty (BPA) is now an increasingly used therapy for patients with surgically inaccessible and residual CTEPH. BPA consistently improves functional status and hemodynamics in such patients and reduces the need for pulmonary vasodilators in follow-up.
- Pulmonary artery denervation (PADN) is currently an investigational therapy showing promise in the treatment of precapillary PH. PADN is currently not available for routine clinical use.
- Balloon atrial septostomy is another interventional therapy that can be used to palliate advanced right heart failure and may be used as a bridge toward definitive management such as lung transplantation.

INTRODUCTION

Disease states resulting in pulmonary hypertension (PH) share the finding of mean pulmonary artery pressure (mPAP) greater than 20 mm Hg,[1] diagnostic criterion set by the sixth world symposium on PH. Within this wide spectrum of PH, 5 separate etiologic groups of PH are described, encompassing anatomic sites of involvement, comorbid conditions, and hemodynamic features (Table 1). Accordingly, therapies for PH also vary by etiologic group and are largely directed toward managing the underlying etiology.[2] Patients with group 1 pulmonary arterial hypertension (PAH) are managed with pulmonary vasodilators. These medications typically act on nitric oxide, prostacyclin, or endothelin signaling pathways leading to pulmonary vasodilatation.[3,4] Recent clinical investigation also shows efficacy in targeting the BMPR-II pathways.[5] Patients with groups 2 and 3 PH are largely managed with therapies targeting underlying left heart and pulmonary parenchymal diseases, respectively. Patients with group 4 PH, also known as chronic thromboembolic PH (CTEPH), are managed with pulmonary endarterectomy (PEA) for those who are surgical candidates, others are traditionally managed with pulmonary vasodilators. Although certainly a step forward biologically, targeted therapies can present financial difficulties. Annual pharmacy costs are estimated at $38,000 among group 1 PH patients in the United States.[6] Additional, adverse effects of the medical therapies

---

[a] Division of Cardiology (Frankel Cardiovascular Center), Department of Internal Medicine, University of Michigan Medical School, 1500 East, Medical Center Drive, SPC 5860, Ann Arbor, MI 48109, USA; [b] Division of Cardiovascular Medicine, North Shore-Long Island Jewish Medical Centers, Northwell Health, Zucker School of Medicine, 270-05 76th Avenue, New Hyde Park, NY 11040, USA
* Corresponding author. 1500 E Medical Center Drive, SPC 5856, Ann Arbor, MI, 48109.
E-mail address: aggarwav@med.umich.edu

Intervent Cardiol Clin 11 (2022) 293–305
https://doi.org/10.1016/j.iccl.2022.01.006
2211-7458/22/Published by Elsevier Inc.

Table 1
Summary of the 5 etiologic groups of pulmonary hypertension

Groups	Key Features	Site of Pulmonary Vasculature Involved	Hemodynamic Findings	Frequency[a] Among Adult Patients with PH[2]
1	*Pulmonary arterial hypertension:* Heritable, idiopathic, drug/toxin-induced, connective tissue related, etc	Precapillary	mPAP > 20 mm Hg PAWP≤15 mm Hg PVR≥3 WU	13.8%
2	*Left heart-related conditions:* Heart failure, valvular disease	a. Isolated postcapillary PH b. Combined precapillary and postcapillary PH	mPAP > 20 mm Hg PAWP > 15 mm Hg PVR – variable	68.5%
3	*Pulmonary related conditions:* Obstructive lung disease, restrictive lung disease, chronic hypoxia	Precapillary	mPAP > 20 mm Hg PAWP≤15 mm Hg PVR≥3 WU	47.0%
4	*Chronic thromboembolic pulmonary disease:* CTEPH Rarely other arterial obstructive pathologies (eg, angiosarcoma)	Precapillary	mPAP > 20 mm Hg PAWP≤15 mm Hg PVR≥3 WU	9.0%
5	*Unclear mechanism:* hematologic disorders, systemic disorders, complex congenital heart disease	Pre, post, or combined PH	mPAP > 20 mm Hg PAWP – variable PVR – variable	

mPAP, mean pulmonary artery pressure; PAWP, pulmonary artery wedge pressure; PVR, pulmonary vascular resistance; WU, woods units.

[a] Multiple etiologic groups may be found in an individual patient, that is, both left heart and pulmonary diseases.

may limit utility in some patients. Traditionally, surgical therapies for PH are limited to PEA for CTEPH patients with proximal disease, and lung transplantation for medically refractory disease. Of patients who do receive lung transplant, 1-year survival is 71.1%,[7] the lowest survival of any patient group undergoing lung transplant.

Such limitations in current PH treatment modalities have raised an interest in finding other novel approaches to durably treat PH. Interventional approaches are being investigated for application to PH (Table 2). Balloon pulmonary angioplasty (BPA) and pulmonary sympathetic denervation are two newer approaches with encouraging early results. Atrial septostomy techniques are also being refined in the role of palliation or bridging to definitive therapy. In this article, we will summarize the current role of interventional therapies for PH and discuss future directions for investigation.

BALLOON PULMONARY ANGIOPLASTY

Patients with group 4 PH, or CTEPH, have occlusions of pulmonary artery branches due to fibrotic reorganization of chronic thrombi. Surgical PEA was the initial therapy available to

Table 2
Major available and investigational interventional approaches for pulmonary hypertension, and the mechanism of therapeutic effect.

Interventional Approach	Balloon Pulmonary Angioplasty	Pulmonary Artery Denervation	Balloon Atrial Septostomy
Implicated mechanism of pulmonary hypertension	Fibrosis of chronic thrombus, obstructing pulmonary artery lumen	Elevated sympathetic tone in pulmonary artery	Progressive RV failure due to end-stage PH, results in LV under filling and low cardiac output
Effect of intervention	Recanalization of pulmonary artery branches, reducing V/Q mismatch, and reducing RV afterload.	Reduced sympathetic tone and pulmonary vasoconstriction, possible reduction in arterial media thickness	Right-to-left shunt leads to reduced RA pressures and facilitates improved LV filling. LV filling results in increased cardiac output.

(Illustrations adapted from Gurevich et al 2020, with permission).

CTEPH patients, though it is limited to suitable operative candidates with surgically accessible disease in main, lobar, or occasionally proximal segmental branches of the pulmonary artery.[8] Registry data suggest that up to 40% of CTEPH patients do not have surgically accessible disease.[9,10] To address this subgroup of nonoperative candidates, BPA has been a therapy under development. BPA is a percutaneous procedure performed over multiple sessions to revascularize previously occluded distal pulmonary artery branches in CTEPH. Increasing BPA experience suggests percutaneous intervention can be a viable therapeutic approach in CTEPH patients who are not candidates for PEA.

HISTORICAL PERSPECTIVE

The first case report of BPA in literature dates back to 1988, in a patient with extensive pulmonary arterial stenoses following prior pulmonary embolism. The patient underwent treatment to 4 total stenotic areas over 3 sessions. His mean PA pressure was reduced from 46 to 35 mm Hg.[11] The authors noted a reperfusion pulmonary edema syndrome following 2 BPA sessions. Next, in 2001, Feinstein and colleagues reported a case series of 18 CTEPH patients managed with pulmonary angioplasty. A mean PA pressure reduction of 9.3 mm Hg was achieved. However, 11 of the 18 patients developed reperfusion pulmonary edema, and 3 patients required mechanical ventilation.[12] Owing to high adverse event rates in these early experiences, BPA was never widely adopted until a renewed approach over the past decade promoted more widespread adoption of the technique.

REFINED APPROACH TO BPA

Mizoguchi and Matsubara and colleagues[13] described their refined approach to BPA in 2012 with a goal to reduce complications from the procedure. The approach suggested careful balloon sizing and incorporated intravascular ultrasound (IVUS) imaging to better characterize vessel size and guide angioplasty balloon selection. The case series of 68 patients reported an average mPAP reduction of 21.4 mm Hg. Forty-one of 68 patients developed reperfusion pulmonary edema and 4 required mechanical ventilation. Following the description of this revised approach, additional centers have reported numerous experiences with BPA. Notable adjunctive approaches described to date in BPA include intraprocedural use of imaging namely IVUS[13] or optical coherence tomography,[14] reperfusion pulmonary edema predictive score,[15] use of pressure measurement to guide angioplasty result,[16] and development of a lesion classification to guide risk stratification for various lesion types seen in CTEPH.[17]

CURRENT EVIDENCE

Khan and colleagues report a meta-analysis and systematic review on 17 noncomparative studies representing 670 CTEPH patients. The analysis found an average mPAP reduction of 14.2 mm Hg, 6MWT improvement of 67.3 m, 1.9% 30-day mortality, and 5.7% long-term mortality.[18] Zoppellaro and colleagues similarly reported on 14 studies representing 725 patients. In their analysis, mPAP was reduced by an average of 10.5 mm Hg, pulmonary vascular resistance (PVR) was decreased by nearly 5 woods units, 6MWT improved by 97 m, and periprocedural mortality was reported at 2.1%. This report also noted complication rates directly related to BPA, with reperfusion pulmonary edema in 9.3%, and other vascular injuries in 2.3% of all BPA sessions. From a clinical guideline standpoint, the 2015 European Society of Cardiology and European Respiratory Society gives a class IIB recommendation that BPA may be considered in patients who are technically nonoperable or carry an unfavorable risk: benefit ratio for PEA.[19]

RECOMMENDED PROCEDURAL APPROACH

Despite numerous reported methods to optimize BPA, a consensus on optimal procedural approach remains elusive. At our institution, the approach to BPA is as follows. First and foremost, patient selection is paramount. All patients suspected to have CTEPH undergo extensive workup, followed by a multidisciplinary case review for PEA or BPA candidacy. BPA procedure should not be performed in isolation and every patient should be first considered for PEA at an expert PAH center.

Once a decision is made to proceed with BPA, interventional planning using non-selective invasive pulmonary angiography, dual-energy CT perfusion imaging and/or ventilation-perfusion scanning identifies target perfusion zones. Such targeting can minimize session count as well as reduce the risk of complications. Most patients still end up needing 4 to 6 BPA sessions in our experience. We believe appropriately targeting perfusion zones reduces the risk of reperfusion edema.

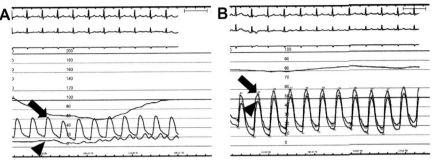

Fig. 1. Pressure wire waveforms before (A) and after (B) balloon pulmonary angioplasty. Following BPA, the distal pressure waveform has become arterialized. Arrow = PA pressure waveform proximal to lesion. Arrowhead = PA pressure waveform distal to lesion. Note: The background scale on the before and after tracings is not equal (0–200 in A, 0–100 in B).

We recommend femoral vein access for BPA, but reports from others have suggested internal jugular vein as an alternative procedure access site. All patients undergo baseline right heart catheterization to assess hemodynamics prior to BPA intervention. Various different coronary guiding catheters are used to selectively engage individual segments in the lung and initial subselective angiography is performed in orthogonal planes to better delineate disease severity. Presence of brisk venous return is considered a very important marker of adequate segmental perfusion.

Once hypoperfusion zones are identified, the next step is to identify pulmonary artery segmental, and subsegmental branches that are likely supplying the affected zone. We recommend using workhorse non-hydrophilic 0.014″ coronary guidewires supported by a balloon catheter and/or guide extension catheter for lesion crossing. Depending on lesion severity, a pressure gradient assessment across the lesion may be helpful to identify parts of the segmental branch that have intraluminal webbing, which can be hard to identify with angiography alone in some cases.

Once diseased vessel lesions are identified and a guidewire is successfully placed across them, angioplasty is initially performed with an undersized compliant balloon. Larger balloons can be used to adequately dilate the lesion in the same session or subsequent sessions. The most important marker of adequate balloon dilatation is the presence of brisk venous return in the perfusion zone of interest on subselective angiography, and arterialization of distal pressure gradient may be informative as well, when performed (Figs. 1 and 2). We set a contrast limit of 3X GFR for BPA at our center and do not use subtraction angiography for subselective angiograms during BPA. Patients are admitted overnight for observation. We perform 2 sessions over 7 days and then repeat sessions the following month. Box 1 summarizes our recommended approach to BPA.

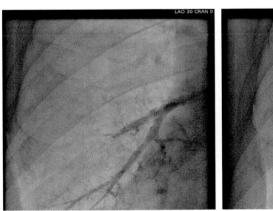
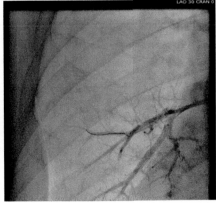

Fig. 2. Resolution of stenotic CTEPH lesion via balloon pulmonary angioplasty, as demonstrated by contrast angiography. Angiograms are taken from before and after BPA.

Box 1
Summary of approach to BPA

Patient Selection

- Multidisciplinary team review at an expert PAH center with surgical expertise for PEA confirms distal, surgically inaccessible disease.

BPA session preparation and guidance

- Treated lesions in any given session should be limited to a unilateral lung (option to selectively intubate contralateral lung in the event of a complication).
- Contrast limit—3x GFR. Radiation limit—2 Gy

Key steps in BPA session

Setup

- Femoral venous access—more readily facilitates catheter delivery into pulmonary segments. Internal jugular vein can be reserved as alternative sites
- Baseline right heart hemodynamics are obtained
- 7 Fr long sheath 70 to 90 cm in length is placed into the right or left main pulmonary artery
- Intravenous unfractionated heparin is given to a goal activated clotting time (ACT) of 200 to 250 seconds

Following lesion site confirmation

- Instrumentation of target vessels performed during breath-hold using coronary guiding catheters.
- Guide extension catheter is sometimes needed to selectively engage segment of interest.
- Workhorse nonhydrophilic soft tip 0.014″ wires supported by a catheter are used to cross lesion
- Baseline pressure measurement performed in selected cases where angiography is not conclusive for an intraluminal web-like lesion.

Angioplasty

- Initial dilatation is performed using undersized balloons and the lesion is sequentially and carefully dilated using larger balloons during the same session or in a staged fashion.
- Intravascular imaging and postpressure gradient measurement are used as adjunctive strategies in selected cases.
- Selective angiography demonstrating the presence of brisk venous return in the perfusion zone of interest is the best marker for adequate dilatation.

Postprocedural care

- Overnight observation
- We recommend a repeat right heart catheterization to reassess hemodynamic improvement 3 months after the last BPA session.

COMPLICATIONS

Pulmonary vascular injury and reperfusion pulmonary edema are the most worrisome complications from BPA. Box 2 describes the current reported incidence and management strategies for these complications.[18,20,21] Vascular injury is often wire or balloon mediated. Most patients develop scant hemoptysis, which resolves with reversal of anticoagulation and supplemental oxygen. More severe injury/perforation occurs more infrequently and often needs intraprocedural coil embolization, plug closure, and/or covered stent placement.[22] Reperfusion pulmonary edema is another common complication during BPA. Grades of severity range from asymptomatic radiographic pulmonary edema to severe respiratory failure requiring intubation and mechanical ventilation. Ejiri and colleagues report high baseline mPAP as an important risk factor for reperfusion pulmonary edema.[23]

Other complications with BPA include cardiac perforation, contrast-induced renal injury, radiation injury, and access site complications.

Box 2
Complications of BPA and management strategies

Reperfusion pulmonary edema

Incidence:

Phan and colleagues 2018—22% mild-moderate, 1.9% severe; Khan and colleagues 2019—16%; Zoppellaro and colleagues—9.3%

Management:

- Supplemental oxygen, noninvasive ventilation as initial support
- Invasive mechanical ventilation as the last measure

Vascular injury

Incidence:

Phan and colleagues 2018—6.8%; Khan and colleagues 2019—3.6%; Zoppellaro and colleagues 2019—2.3%

Supportive maneuvers:

- Supplemental oxygen, or noninvasive ventilation
- Turn patient on their side to place proceduralized lung downwards
- Selective single lung intubation to ventilate nonhemorrhagic lung

Hemorrhage control maneuvers:

- Immediate balloon tamponade of vessel
- Reversal of anticoagulation
- Covered stent implantation
- Gelfoam injection
- Coil embolization
- Vascular plug closure

FUTURE DIRECTIONS

Contemporary BPA is a safe and viable interventional therapy for distal inoperable CTEPH. Key next steps include the development of a consensus approach and standardization to best optimize clinical outcomes. We additionally await the results of randomized clinical trials comparing BPA to medical therapy with riociguat. The RACE (riociguat vs balloon pulmonary Angioplasty in nonoperable chronic thromboembolic pulmonary hypertension; NCT02634203) and MR-BPA (multicenter randomized controlled trial based on BPA for chronic thromboembolic PH; UMIN00001 9549) trials will be instructive in clinically guiding utilization of BPA procedures.

PULMONARY ARTERY DENERVATION

Pulmonary artery denervation (PADN) is another therapy that is starting to show promise in early investigation in a wide variety of PH subgroups.

HISTORIC AND PHYSIOLOGIC BASIS

Prior studies have demonstrated a role for sympathetic nervous system overactivation in the pathogenesis of PH.[24–26] The degree of sympathetic nervous system overactivation appears related to PH disease severity.[27] The goal of sympathetic nerve ablation is to reduce afferent and efferent sympathetic nerve signaling involved in baroreceptor reflex-related vasoconstriction of the pulmonary arteries.[28] Catheter-based interventions targeting sympathetic nerves are not new, as numerous studies have investigated the efficacy of various renal artery denervation strategies for systemic hypertension.[29]

Early animal studies of PADN demonstrated histologic changes in the pulmonary arteries and favorable biochemical changes within the adventitial nerves.[30] Canine studies have demonstrated sustained sympathetic nerve effects following denervation, including reduction of pulmonary artery medial wall thickness, and improved hemodynamics.[31]

EARLY HUMAN EXPERIENCES

Following encouraging animal studies, Chen and colleagues reported a first-in-human experience with PADN in 2013. This study included 13 patients with PAH, reporting an average mPAP improvement of 19 mm Hg and a mean 6MWT improvement of 167 m at 3 months follow-up.[32] This study was met with skepticism. Notable critiques included the pathophysiologic basis upon which PADN was proposed, the atypical patient population for PAH, and medication withdrawals during the study period.[33] In a subsequent study, Chen and colleagues published a 66 patient series of PADN, with 1-year follow-up demonstrating mPAP reduction of 8.5 mm Hg. In this phase II study, Chen and colleagues[34] reported zero PADN procedural complications, progressive PAH-related events in 15% of patients, and 12% all-cause deaths in the 1-year follow-up interval.

CURRENT EVIDENCE

Since the initial single-center studies, additional experiences with PADN have been reported in the literature (Table 3). The TROPHY-1 multicenter single-arm study of therapeutic IVUS PADN included 23 PAH patients treated with dual oral or triple nonparenteral therapy. At 4 or 6 months follow-up, PVR was 17.8% reduced on average.[35] Among the 23 patients, no procedure-related serious adverse events were noted. To further evaluate the safety and efficacy of ultrasound PADN, the TROPHY-PAH Pivotal study (TReatment of Pulmonary HYpertension for PAH Pivotal Study; NCT04570228) is expected as a randomized, sham-controlled trial in the coming years. In addition to PADN studies in PAH patients, other studies summarized in Table 3 have included patients with groups 2, 3, or 4 PH. As PADN remains an investigational therapy, it is currently not available for routine clinical use outside of clinical trials.

PROCEDURAL APPROACH FOR PADN

Reports to date largely describe the use of radiofrequency ablation catheters or high-energy endovascular ultrasound for PADN. In both approaches, the catheters are delivered to the main PA from a peripheral vein. Rothman and colleagues[28] report anatomic mapping of pulmonary artery innervation in human cadavers, finding 71% sympathetic fiber predominance, predominantly in main PA trunk greater than left or right PA, at depths ranging from 1 to 12 mm. Based on such anatomic studies, circumferential ablation is generally performed at the main, right, and left pulmonary, with a goal of destroying the sympathetic fibers within adventitia. Although most approaches have involved circumferential ablation, Fujisawa and colleagues[36] reported a selective ablation strategy targeted to areas where high-frequency stimulation would induce bradycardia and thus signify autonomic nerve location.

PALLIATIVE AND BRIDGING MEASURES—ATRIAL SEPTOSTOMY

In cases of refractory PH and progression to right ventricular (RV) failure, interventional approaches to offload the failing RV have been investigated. At this time, atrial septostomy is most commonly performed as a palliation, creating an interatrial right-to-left shunt. This shunt offloads the right heart and improves left ventricle filling. Consequently, cardiac output improves as does overall systemic oxygen delivery, despite a reduced systemic oxygen saturation. Rare cases of percutaneous Potts' shunt between left PA and aorta have also been reported, though with higher incidence of adverse outcomes.[37]

As expected, most reports suggest limited benefit in patients with WHO functional class IV disease with end-stage right heart failure despite medical therapy.[38,39] Khan and colleagues report a meta-analysis of 16 balloon atrial septostomy studies, representing 204 patients. In the analysis, the authors determine that right atrial pressure was reduced by a mean of 2.77 mm Hg, cardiac index improved by 0.62 L/min/m², and mean arterial oxygen saturation was reduced by 8.45%. The pooled incidence of mortality was 4.8% at 48 hours, 14.6% at 30 days, and 37.7% at long-term follow-up.[40] Owing to the relatively high procedure-related mortality and long-term mortality, balloon atrial septostomy is only suited as a bridge to definitive procedures such as lung transplantation and/or last resort palliation in carefully selected patients.

SUMMARY

Research evidence has illustrated biochemical targets for medical treatment of PAH. Although effective, treatment barriers still loom for patients with PH. In addition to targeted pharmacologic therapy, more recent advances have demonstrated pathophysiologic targets from an interventional approach as well. The role of interventional cardiology for adjunctive therapies in PH is under growing investigation.

Percutaneous interventions have shown promise in many areas of cardiovascular disease. PH is no exception to this. Carefully selected

Table 3
Early published experiences with PADN

Study (y)	Study Size, Patient Characteristics	Study Design	Device	Follow-Up Interval	Outcome	Notable Complications & Follow-Up Mortality
Chen et al (2013)[32]	13 patients: All with idiopathic PAH	Nonrandomized, nonblinded controlled phase 1	Dedicated 7.5-F temperature sensing and ablation catheter	3 mo	mPAP: ↓19 mm Hg PVR: −1120 dyne*s*cm^{-5} 6MWT: ↑167 m	
Chen et al (2015)[34]	66 patients: —39 with group 1 disease —18 with group 2 disease —9 with residual group 4 PH despite surgical endarterectomy	Open-label phase II	Dedicated 7-F temperature sensing ablation catheter	12 mo	PVR: ↓4.9 WU 6MWT: ↑94 m	
Zhang et al (2019)[41]	98 patients: All with group 2 PH	Randomized, sham-controlled: —PADN alone vs —Sildenafil with sham PADN	Dedicated 7-F temperature sensing ablation catheter	6 mo	6MWT: —PADN—↑83 m —Sham—↑15 m PVR: —PADN—↓2.2 WU —Sham—↓0.16 WU	PADN group: −3 deaths. At 6d (pump failure), 29d (sudden death), 72d (fatal PE). Sham group: −6 deaths. At 17d (sudden death), 36d (fatal PE), and 17, 93, 100, 154d (pump failure)
Rothman et al (2020)[35]	23 patients with PAH: —8 idiopathic —3 drug-use assoc. —12 CTD related	Open-label, early feasibility study	Intravascular ultrasound	4–6 mo	6MWT: ↑42 m PVR: ↓94 dyne*s*cm^{-5}	No procedure-related adverse events

(continued on next page)

Table 3
(continued)

Study (y)	Study Size, Patient Characteristics	Study Design	Device	Follow-Up Interval	Outcome	Notable Complications & Follow-Up Mortality
Romanov et al (2020)[42]	50 patients: All with residual group 4 PH (CTEPH) after PEA	Randomized, sham-controlled: —PADN alone vs —Riociguat w/sham PADN	RF ablation	12 mo	6MWT: —PADN—↑90 m —Sham—↑19 m PVR: —PADN—↓258 dyne*s*cm^{-5} —Sham—↓149 dyne*s*cm^{-5}	PADN group: —8 periprocedural transient sinus bradycardias or asystolic pause —1 subsequent heart failure hospitalization —1 death Sham: —7 heart failure hospitalizations —2 deaths
Witkowski et al (2021)[43]	10 patients —all with group 2 PH associated with HFrEF	Single-arm study of PADN	RF ablation	6 mo	PVR: ↑1.8 WU (among survivors) 6MWT: ↓7 m (among survivors)	No acute, in-hospital local or systemic complications of PADN 3 deaths due to heart failure

patients with CTEPH can be treated with BPA safely and effectively. For the broader PH population, radiofrequency ablation catheter or IVUS-mediated PADN is being studied as a mechanism to achieve hemodynamic and symptomatic improvement. Finally, palliating or bridging intervention with balloon atrial septostomy can be pursued percutaneously as well. These procedures may show promise for patients when no other therapies are available. Carefully designed and well-powered clinical trials will help define the role of interventional cardiology among the tools used to treat PH.

CLINICS CARE POINTS

- Patients with a prior history of venous thromboembolic disease, persistent dyspnea, and exercise intolerance should be screened for chronic thromboembolic pulmonary hypertension (CTEPH).

- All patients with CTEPH should be evaluated at an expert center with expertise in pulmonary endarterectomy and balloon pulmonary angioplasty.

- Interventional therapies such as BPA should only be offered after multidisciplinary discussion within an expert PAH program.

ACKNOWLEDGMENTS

None

DISCLOSURE

The authors have nothing to disclose.

REFERENCES

1. Simonneau G, Montani D, Celermajer DS, et al. Haemodynamic definitions and updated clinical classification of pulmonary hypertension. Eur Respir J 2019;53:1801913.
2. Wijeratne DT, Lajkosz K, Brogly SB, et al. Increasing incidence and prevalence of world health organization groups 1 to 4 pulmonary hypertension: a population-based cohort study in Ontario, Canada. Circ Cardiovasc Qual Outcomes 2018;11:e003973.
3. Humbert M, Sitbon O, Simonneau G. Treatment of pulmonary arterial hypertension. N Engl J Med 2004;351:1425–36.
4. Galie N, Corris PA, Frost A, et al. Updated treatment algorithm of pulmonary arterial hypertension. J Am Coll Cardiol 2013;62:D60–72.
5. Humbert M, McLaughlin V, Gibbs JSR, et al. Sotatercept for the treatment of pulmonary arterial hypertension. N Engl J Med 2021;384:1204–15.
6. Sikirica M, Iorga SR, Bancroft T, et al. The economic burden of pulmonary arterial hypertension (PAH) in the US on payers and patients. BMC Health Serv Res 2014;14:676.
7. George MP, Champion HC, Pilewski JM. Lung transplantation for pulmonary hypertension. Pulm Circ 2011;1:182–91.
8. Madani MM. Surgical treatment of chronic thromboembolic pulmonary hypertension: Pulmonary thromboendarterectomy. Methodist DeBakey Cardiovasc J 2016;12:213–8.
9. Mayer E, Jenkins D, Lindner J, et al. Surgical management and outcome of patients with chronic thromboembolic pulmonary hypertension: results from an international prospective registry. J Thorac Cardiovasc Surg 2011;141:702–10.
10. Pepke-Zaba J, Delcroix M, Lang I, et al. Chronic thromboembolic pulmonary hypertension (CTEPH): results from an international prospective registry. Circulation 2011;124:1973–81.
11. Voorburg JA, Cats VM, Buis B, et al. Balloon angioplasty in the treatment of pulmonary hypertension caused by pulmonary embolism. Chest 1988;94:1249–53.
12. Feinstein JA, Goldhaber SZ, Lock JE, et al. Balloon pulmonary angioplasty for treatment of chronic thromboembolic pulmonary hypertension. Circulation 2001;103:10–3.
13. Mizoguchi H, Ogawa A, Munemasa M, et al. Refined balloon pulmonary angioplasty for inoperable patients with chronic thromboembolic pulmonary hypertension. Circ Cardiovasc Interv 2012;5:748–55.
14. Sugimura K, Fukumoto Y, Satoh K, et al. Percutaneous transluminal pulmonary angioplasty markedly improves pulmonary hemodynamics and long-term prognosis in patients with chronic thromboembolic pulmonary hypertension. Circ J 2012;76:485–8.
15. Inami T, Kataoka M, Shimura N, et al. Pulmonary edema predictive scoring index (PEPSI), a new index to predict risk of reperfusion pulmonary edema and improvement of hemodynamics in percutaneous transluminal pulmonary angioplasty. JACC Cardiovasc Interv 2013;6:725–36.
16. Inami T, Kataoka M, Shimura N, et al. Pressure-wire-guided percutaneous transluminal pulmonary angioplasty: a breakthrough in catheter-interventional therapy for chronic thromboembolic pulmonary hypertension. JACC Cardiovasc Interv 2014;7:1297–306.
17. Kawakami T, Ogawa A, Miyaji K, et al. Novel angiographic classification of each vascular lesion in chronic thromboembolic pulmonary hypertension

based on selective angiogram and results of balloon pulmonary angioplasty. Circ Cardiovasc Interv 2016;9:e003318.

18. Khan MS, Amin E, Memon MM, et al. Meta-analysis of use of balloon pulmonary angioplasty in patients with inoperable chronic thromboembolic pulmonary hypertension. Int J Cardiol 2019;291:134–9.

19. Galie N, Humbert M, Vachiery JL, et al. 2015 ESC/ERS guidelines for the diagnosis and treatment of pulmonary hypertension: the joint task force for the diagnosis and treatment of pulmonary hypertension of the european society of cardiology (ESC) and the european respiratory society (ERS): endorsed by: association for european paediatric and congenital cardiology (AEPC), international society for heart and lung transplantation (ISHLT). Eur Respir J 2015;46:903–75.

20. Phan K, Jo HE, Xu J, et al. Medical therapy versus balloon angioplasty for CTEPH: a systematic review and meta-analysis. Heart Lung Circ 2018;27:89–98.

21. Zoppellaro G, Badawy MR, Squizzato A, et al. Balloon pulmonary angioplasty in patients with chronic thromboembolic pulmonary hypertension-a systematic review and meta-analysis. Circ J 2019;83:1660–7.

22. Mahmud E, Behnamfar O, Ang L, et al. Balloon pulmonary angioplasty for chronic thromboembolic pulmonary hypertension. Interv Cardiol Clin 2018;7:103–17.

23. Ejiri K, Ogawa A, Fujii S, et al. Vascular injury is a major cause of lung injury after balloon pulmonary angioplasty in patients with chronic thromboembolic pulmonary hypertension. Circ Cardiovasc Interv 2018;11:e005884.

24. Juratsch CE, Jengo JA, Castagna J, et al. Experimental pulmonary hypertension produced by surgical and chemical denervation of the pulmonary vasculature. Chest 1980;77:525–30.

25. Nootens M, Kaufmann E, Rector T, et al. Neurohormonal activation in patients with right ventricular failure from pulmonary hypertension: relation to hemodynamic variables and endothelin levels. J Am Coll Cardiol 1995;26:1581–5.

26. Velez-Roa S, Ciarka A, Najem B, et al. Increased sympathetic nerve activity in pulmonary artery hypertension. Circulation 2004;110:1308–12.

27. Ciarka A, Doan V, Velez-Roa S, et al. Prognostic significance of sympathetic nervous system activation in pulmonary arterial hypertension. Am J Respir Crit Care Med 2010;181:1269–75.

28. Rothman A, Jonas M, Castel D, et al. Pulmonary artery denervation using catheter-based ultrasonic energy. EuroIntervention 2019;15:722–30.

29. Weber MA, Mahfoud F, Schmieder RE, et al. Renal denervation for treating hypertension: current scientific and clinical evidence. JACC Cardiovasc Interv 2019;12:1095–105.

30. Rothman AM, Arnold ND, Chang W, et al. Pulmonary artery denervation reduces pulmonary artery pressure and induces histological changes in an acute porcine model of pulmonary hypertension. Circ Cardiovasc Interv 2015;8:e002569.

31. Zhou L, Zhang J, Jiang XM, et al. Pulmonary artery denervation attenuates pulmonary arterial remodeling in dogs with pulmonary arterial hypertension induced by dehydrogenized monocrotaline. JACC Cardiovasc Interv 2015;8:2013–23.

32. Chen SL, Zhang FF, Xu J, et al. Pulmonary artery denervation to treat pulmonary arterial hypertension: the single-center, prospective, first-in-man PADN-1 study (first-in-man pulmonary artery denervation for treatment of pulmonary artery hypertension). J Am Coll Cardiol 2013;62:1092–100.

33. Galie N, Manes A. New treatment strategies for pulmonary arterial hypertension: hopes or hypes? J Am Coll Cardiol 2013;62:1101–2.

34. Chen SL, Zhang H, Xie DJ, et al. Hemodynamic, functional, and clinical responses to pulmonary artery denervation in patients with pulmonary arterial hypertension of different causes: phase II results from the Pulmonary Artery Denervation-1 study. Circ Cardiovasc Interv 2015;8:e002837.

35. Rothman AMK, Vachiery JL, Howard LS, et al. Intravascular Ultrasound Pulmonary Artery Denervation to Treat Pulmonary Arterial Hypertension (TROPHY1): Multicenter, Early Feasibility Study. JACC Cardiovasc Interv 2020;13:989–99.

36. Fujisawa T, Kataoka M, Kawakami T, et al. Pulmonary artery denervation by determining targeted ablation sites for treatment of pulmonary arterial hypertension. Circ Cardiovasc Interv 2017;10:e005812.

37. Bobhate P, Mohanty SR, Tailor K, et al. Potts shunt as an effective palliation for patients with end stage pulmonary arterial hypertension. Indian Heart J 2021;73:196–204.

38. Sandoval J, Gaspar J, Pulido T, et al. Graded balloon dilation atrial septostomy in severe primary pulmonary hypertension. J Am Coll Cardiol 1998;32:297–304.

39. Kurzyna M, Dabrowski M, Bielecki D, et al. Atrial septostomy in treatment of end-stage right heart failure in patients with pulmonary hypertension. Chest 2007;131:977–83.

40. Khan MS, Memon MM, Amin E, et al. Use of balloon atrial septostomy in patients with advanced pulmonary arterial hypertension: a systematic review and meta-analysis. Chest 2019;156:53–63.

41. Zhang H, Zhang J, Chen M, et al. Pulmonary artery denervation significantly increases 6-min walk distance for patients with combined pre- and post-capillary pulmonary hypertension associated with

left heart failure: the PADN-5 study. JACC Cardiovasc Interv 2019;12:274–84.

42. Romanov A, Cherniavskiy A, Novikova N, et al. Pulmonary artery denervation for patients with residual pulmonary hypertension after pulmonary endarterectomy. J Am Coll Cardiol 2020;76: 916–26.

43. Witkowski A, Szumowski L, Urbanek P, et al. Transcatheter pulmonary denervation in patients with left heart failure with reduced ejection fraction and combined precapillary and postcapillary pulmonary hypertension: A prospective single center experience. Catheter Cardiovasc Interv 2021;98(3): 588–94.

The Clinical Problem of Pelvic Venous Disorders

Abu Baker Sheikh, MD[a], Marat Fudim, MD, MHS[b,c,*], Ishan Garg, MBBS[a],
Abdul Mannan Khan Minhas, MD[d], Asher A. Sobotka[e], Manesh R. Patel, MD[b,c],
Marvin H. Eng, MD[f], Paul A. Sobotka, MD[g,*]

KEYWORDS

- Pelvic venous disorders • Pelvic congestion syndrome • Nutcracker syndrome
- May-Thurner syndrome • Cardiovenous syndrome • Percutaneous embolization
- Percutaneous stenting

KEY POINTS

- Pelvic venous disorders represent a group of inter-related pathologic conditions that is grossly underdiagnosed.
- Pelvic venous disorders can present with a wide range of pelvic, urinary, lower extremity, and cardiac symptoms.
- Pelvic venous disorders clinical symptoms are based on the route of transmission of venous hypertension to interconnected venous reservoirs.
- Imaging (with ultrasound examination, computed tomography scans, and MRI) is essential for diagnosis and guiding management.
- Percutaneous interventions (embolization and stenting) are a safe and effective treatment option.

INTRODUCTION

Pelvic venous disorder (PeVD) causes multiple clinically debilitating symptoms but is grossly underdiagnosed.[1-4] In 1 study, 45% of patients with chronic pelvic pain (CPP) had an underlying PeVD.[1] CPP is defined as noncyclical pain in the lower abdomen and pelvis that lasts longer than 6 months.[5] CPP affects millions of women and accounts for nearly 40% of all gynecologic visits; however, an accurate diagnosis is made in only one-half of these cases.[6] It is estimated that PeVDs are responsible for approximately one-third of cases and are second only to endometriosis as a cause of CPP.[3] A high prevalence of asymptomatic PeVD (40%–60%) has also been noted in women undergoing cross-sectional computed tomography (CT) scans or MRIs.[2]

PeVD includes all chronic disorders of pelvic veins that are caused by venous retrograde flow and hypertension in the pelvic veins.[4,6] It encompasses a large spectrum of morphologic and functional abnormalities of the pelvic venous system, which may or may not be symptomatic. PeVD can often present with a range of overlapping pelvic, urinary, lower extremity, and cardiac symptoms.[3]

Historically, these disorders were classified into syndromes (based on symptoms) such as pelvic congestion syndrome, nutcracker syndrome (NCS), and May-Thurner syndrome (MTS). This syndromic nomenclature undermines our understanding and management of complex inter-related

[a] Department of Internal Medicine, University of New Mexico Health Sciences Center, 1021 Medical Arts Avenue NE, Albuquerque, NM 87102, USA; [b] Division of Cardiology, Duke University Medical Center, 200 Trent Drive, Durham, NC 27710, USA; [c] Duke Clinical Research Institute, 300 West Morgan Street, Durham, NC 27701, USA; [d] Department of Internal Medicine, Forrest General Hospital, 6051 US 49, Hattiesburg, MS 39401, USA; [e] University of Pennsylvania, Philadelphia, PA 19104, USA; [f] Division of Cardiology, University of Arizona, Banner University Medical Center, 1111 E McDowell Rd, Phoenix, AZ 85006, USA; [g] The Ohio State University, 281 West Lane Avenue, Columbus, OH 43210, USA
* Corresponding authors.
E-mail addresses: Marat.fudim@duke.edu (M.F.); paul.a.sobotka@gmail.com (P.A.S.)

pathophysiology involved in these disorders. However, several authors and multidisciplinary panels have recently advocated for adopting a single term, PeVD, unifying these related conditions' causes and clinical consequences.[4,7,8]

The purpose of this article is to review the (1) underlying anatomical pathophysiology, (2) potential clinical presentations, and (3) a diagnostic and treatment approach with a focus on current interventional percutaneous treatment options.

PELVIC VENOUS ANATOMY
Drainage Pathway

The pelvic venous drainage consists of 3 interconnected systems: the left renal and ovarian and gonadal veins, the iliac veins (common, external, and internal), and the lower extremity veins (Fig. 1). PeVD is caused by venous reflux and/or obstruction, alone or in various combinations in these vein segments (Fig. 2). The internal iliac vein drains venous blood from the pelvic viscera, the walls of the pelvis, the gluteal region, and the perineum. The external iliac vein is a continuation of the femoral vein (which drains the lower extremity) when the femoral vein crosses underneath the inguinal ligament. The ovarian venous plexus drains into the ipsilateral gonadal vein, which, on the left, drains into the left renal vein and, on the right, drains directly into the inferior vena cava (IVC)[9,10] (see Fig. 1).

It is also important to note that there can be several normal variants in pelvic venous anatomy, including internal iliac veins that drain into the contralateral common iliac vein or duplicated IVCs.[11,12]

Valves

Venous valves maintain the 1-way flow of blood back to the heart. A lack of and incompetent vein valves play a pivotal role in the

development of PeVD. The internal iliac veins, distal tributaries (90% of the cases), and pelvic venous plexuses are valveless.[9,10] In the ovarian vein, valves are absent in 15% of women. However, ovarian vein valves, when present, are incompetent in up to 40% of cases.[13,14]

Pelvic Escape Points

It is also important to note that distal tributaries of the internal iliac vein (from the uterus, ovaries, bladder, and parietal structures of the pelvis) communicate inferiorly through the pelvic floor (pelvic escape points) with the superficial veins of the proximal lower extremity and vulva via the internal pudendal, obturator, round ligament (inguinal) and inferior gluteal veins.[4,15–17]

A combination of lack of or incompetent venous valves, and the presence of escape points, means that venous hypertension from reflux or obstruction can be transmitted to the adjacent or more caudal venous reservoirs. For example, venous hypertension in the internal iliac vein can be transmitted to the lower extremity and vulvar veins through escape points, leading to distention (varices) of these venous reservoirs.[15,16] Therefore, based on the pattern of transmission of this venous hypertension to adjacent and/or distal venous reservoirs, different clinical symptoms can be seen with the same primary pathophysiology and vice versa (different primary pathophysiology can result in similar clinical symptoms).

PELVIC VENOUS DISORDERCLASSIFICATION

The Clinical–Etiology–Anatomy–Pathophysiology (CEAP) classification is the most widely used classification system for lower extremity chronic venous disorders. This standardized reporting

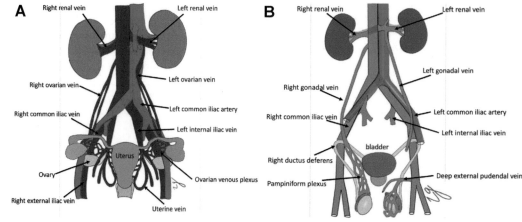

Fig. 1. An illustrative diagram shows the normal pelvic venous system. (*A*) Female. (*B*) Male.

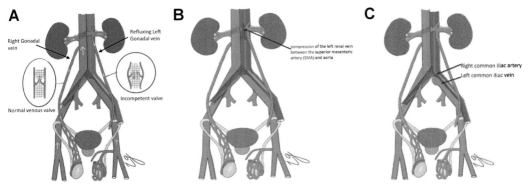

Fig. 2. Common causes of PeVDs. (*A*) Incompetent gonadal vein valves. *Arrows* show venous blood flow, with reversal of venous blood flow (reflux) in the left gonadal vein owing to an incompetent venous valve. A normal venous valve can be noted in the right gonadal vein for comparison. (*B*) NCS, caused by compression of the left renal vein between the superior mesenteric artery and aorta (anterior NCS). (*C*) MTS, caused by compression of left common iliac vein between the right common iliac artery and vertebral body.

method was developed to serve as a systematic guide in the daily clinical investigation of patients as an orderly documentation system and basis for decisions regarding appropriate treatment.

Based on similar principles, the American Vein Lymphatic Society in 2021 proposed a new classification based on symptoms (S), varices (V), and complex anatomic–pathophysiology (P). The clinical symptoms (S) domain is determined by subscripts ranging from 0 to 3. The varices (V) domain is determined by the site of varices: the (i) renal hilum, (ii) venous plexuses of the pelvis, and (iii) extrapelvic vessels of pelvic origin. The pathophysiology (P) domain includes pelvic and abdominal vein anatomy (A), symptom-related hemodynamic abnormalities (H), and underlying etiology (E) subfields. Anatomic parts of the abdomen and pelvis (PA) are indicated with anatomic abbreviations. Hemodynamic (PH) irregularities are indicated by reflux (R), obstruction (O), or both (R, O). The etiology (PE) is indicated with thrombotic (T), nonthrombotic (NT), or congenital (C). All 3 components are indicated by a subscript in the "P" category. According to this classification, the pelvic disease score of an individual is shown as $SVP_{A,H,E}$. The authors hoped that this classification system would help to improve clinical decision-making, physician communication, the development of disease-specific outcome measures, and identifying homogenous patient populations for clinical trials.[7,8]

ETIOLOGY OF PELVIC VENOUS DISORDERS

A combination of environmental, anatomic, medical, and genetic risk factors causing venous valvular incompetence and/or obstruction (intrinsic and extrinsic) can contribute to the development of PeVD. Causes of pelvic venous internal obstruction include acute or chronic resolving clots within the pelvic veins and extending to the IVC, MTS, and NCS.[18]

The causes of extrinsic obstruction include tumor, fibrosis owing to prior surgery, radiation, chronic inflammatory bowel disease, prior trauma, arterial compression of adjacent veins, and entrapment between bony, ligament, tendons, or pelvic fat.[19–23] Pregnancy itself is a form of extrinsic pelvic vein compression associated with both venous hypertension and exercise intolerance linked to impaired venous return and oxygenation, and intermittent complete IVC obstruction with position is a frequent cause of hypertension in pregnancy.[24]

With an increasing incidence and high prevalence worldwide, obesity (defined as a body mass index of 30 kg/m^2) is an important risk factor for the development of PeVD.[25–28] Obesity (especially visceral) can lead to an increase in intra-abdominal pressure (9–14 mm Hg in obese vs 5–7 mm Hg in nonobese individuals), resulting in extrinsic pelvic vein compression.[29,30]

In addition, various genetic mutations such as TIE2, NOTCH3, thrombomodulin, type 2 transforming growth factor- β, and FOXC2 have also been linked with the development of PeVD.[31] Irrespective of the underlying etiology, the main pathogenic pathway is similar to what is seen in the development of deep vein thrombosis (DVT), that is, a combination of (1) venous stasis, (2) activation of blood coagulation, and (3) vein damage. For instance, prolonged venous stasis and venous hypertension can lead to increased expression of matrix metalloproteinases, causing disruption of vein wall (endothelium and smooth muscle) integrity. This endothelial injury, in turn, can activate inflammatory cascade and leukocyte infiltration resulting in chronic venous distention and reflux (retrograde flow).[32,33]

Here we discuss the most commonly noted etiologies, including incompetent gonadal vein valves, NTS, and MTS (see Fig. 2).

Incompetent Gonadal Vein Valves

Incompetent gonadal vein valves are one the most commonly identified cause of PeVD. It can be both acquired or congenital. Studies have noted that even though gonadal veins are present in 85% to 90% of the individuals (more frequently absent in the left gonadal vein), they are incompetent in more than 40% of these individuals. Pregnancy (venous distention and extrinsic compression) is the most common cause of acquired gonadal vein valve incompetence. This partly explains why PeVD is more frequently seen in multiparous women[34] (see Fig. 2).

Nutcracker Syndrome and Renal Vein Entrapment Syndrome

NCS is a form of extrinsic venous compression disorder. It was first reported in 1950 by El-Sadr and Mina and later named by de Schepper in 1972.[35,36] NCS is characterized by compression of the left renal vein between the superior mesenteric artery and aorta (anterior NCS) (see Fig. 2). In some individuals with anatomic variants, the left renal vein can be retroaortic (3% of cases) or circumaortic (17% of cases).[37] In the retroaortic variant, the left renal vein is compressed between the aorta and vertebral body (posterior NCS).[38] However, posterior NCS is rare, noted in only 0.5% to 3.7% of cases.[39] Individuals with a lower body mass index are at an increased risk for developing NCS, because a lack of mesenteric fat padding can lead to a decrease in aortic–superior mesenteric artery angle. Similarly, individuals with a steeper aortic–superior mesenteric artery angle and a higher set left renal vein are at an increased risk for NCS.[39] The exact prevalence of NCS is unknown, partly owing to the lack of standardized diagnostic criteria.[40,41] It is also important to note that asymptomatic nutcracker anatomy (also known as the nutcracker phenomenon) can be seen as an incidental finding in cross-sectional imaging in 2% to 18% of patients.[42,43] It usually presents with hematuria (secondary to hemorrhage from thin-walled varices into the renal calyceal fornices), orthostatic proteinuria, and flank pain. However, based on venous hypertension escape pathways, it can present with symptoms similar to any other PeVD.[35]

May-Thurner Syndrome and Cockett Syndrome

MTS is also a form of extrinsic venous compression disorder caused by compression of the left common iliac vein between the right common iliac artery and vertebral body (usually L5)[44] (see Fig. 2). Multiple variants have been reported, including right-sided venous compression in patients with a left-sided IVC and compression of the IVC by the right common iliac artery.[45,46] Chronic compression can lead to intimal proliferation and fibrosis, subsequently leading to the formation of internal bands and venous obstruction.[47]

Like NTS, there are no standardized diagnostic criteria for MTS. The exact prevalence of MTS is unknown. Although multiple studies have noted a significant hemodynamic compression owing to MTS in 22% to 50% of people, only a few patients develop a symptomatic disease.[48–52] MTS is most commonly seen in young females in their third or fourth decade after prolonged immobility, pregnancy, or hormonal contraception. Symptomatic MTS usually manifests as thromboembolism (DVT) and worsening stenosis.[52,53]

CLINICAL FEATURES OF PELVIC VENOUS DISORDERS

PeVD can present with a spectrum of signs and symptoms. The relationship between pelvic venous pathology and clinical features can be very complex. Similar underlying primary abnormality can present with different symptoms and vice versa. To simplify the correlation between underlying pathophysiology and clinical symptoms, some authors have suggested that clinical symptoms should be divided based on involved venous reservoirs. The pelvic venous drainage can be divided into 3 interconnected series of "venous blood reservoirs," namely, renal/ovarian, common/internal iliac, and lower extremity veins.[3,54–56] The clinical feature of any PeVD depends on which reservoirs the venous hypertension is transmitted to.[57] For example, primary ovarian/internal iliac reflux can present with predominant pelvic symptoms (owing to distension of the pelvic venous system, if uncompensated) or predominately lower extremity symptoms (varices, edema) (if compensated, owing to decompression via collaterals into lower extremity venous reservoirs) (Fig. 3).

CPP and pelvic origin lower extremity varicose veins are the 2 most commonly seen presentations in women. Sulakvelidze and colleagues,[58] in a study on presentation patterns

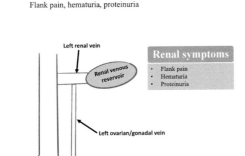

Flank pain, hematuria, proteinuria

Fig. 3. Clinical features of PeVDs depend on whether the increase in the pressure is directly transmitted to the distal venous reservoir (uncompensated reflux or obstruction) or decompressed into more caudal reservoirs by associated collaterals (compensated reflux or obstruction).

in women with PeVDs, noted that pelvic and leg symptoms were inversely related to age, with the lowest prevalence of PeVD in patients in their 20s.

Based on this premise, the major clinical presentations seen in PeVD patients are:

A. Pelvic symptoms—CPP and perineal varicosities
B. Renal symptoms—flank pain, hematuria, and proteinuria
C. Extrapelvic symptoms—lower extremity varicose veins, swelling, venous claudication, and vulvar varicosities
D. Systemic symptoms—heart failure, unexplained pulmonary emboli, and post-thrombotic syndrome

Pelvic Symptoms
Chronic pelvic pain
The American College of Obstetrics & Gynecology defines CPP as constant or intermittent pain from the pelvic organs or other pelvic structures that persists for at least 6 months and results in functional disability or requirements for medical care.[54] CPP affects millions of women and accounts for nearly 40% of all gynecologic visits. In addition, CPP can result in debilitating limitations in physical, emotional, and work-related functional capacity. CPP has an extensive list of potential causes, including endometriosis, irritable bowel syndrome, interstitial cystitis, myofascial pelvic pain, central and peripheral sensitization, depression, and generalized anxiety disorders.[54,59,60] However, it is important not to overlook PeVD as one of the potential

causes. Although the exact prevalence of PeVD in women with CPP is unknown, 1 study involving 148 consecutive patients undergoing evaluation for CPP found that 43% of women had PeVD. A solitary diagnosis of PeVD was made in 31%; by comparison, a solitary diagnoses of endometriosis and postoperative scarring were made in 39% and 11% patients, respectively[61] (**Fig. 4**).

The CPP is usually exacerbated with standing or at the end of the day, during menses (potentially owing to higher level of estrogen), and can be associated with dyspareunia, bloating, back pain, dysmenorrhea, vulvar varicosities, lower extremity varicosities, and renal symptoms.[62] On physical examination, tenderness at the ovarian point (a point one-third of the way between the umbilicus and the anterior superior iliac spine) and extreme pain on gentle bimanual examination of the ovary and surrounding tissues with history of postcoital ache, dyspareunia in a menstruating woman is highly sensitive and specific for PeVD.[63]

Interestingly, CPP owing to PeVD is not seen in men, primarily owing to the extrapelvic course of gonadal veins and different arrangements of pelvic venous plexuses compared with women.[64,65]

Testicular Varicocele
A testicular varicocele is an abnormal dilation and enlargement of the scrotal venous pampiniform plexus, which drains blood from each testicle (see **Fig. 4**). It is seen in approximately 15% of the adult male population and 35% of men with primary infertility.[66] It is usually

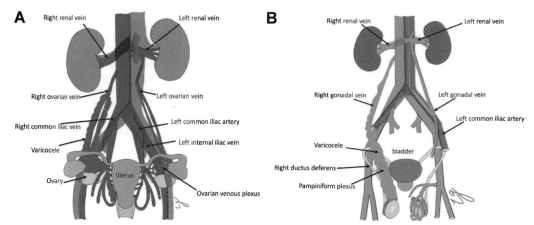

Fig. 4. An illustrative diagram showing common pelvic symptoms of PeVDs. (*A*) CPP (owing to pelvic venous congestion). (*B*) Testicular varicocele.

asymptomatic, but can also present with testicular pain, infertility, and testicular atrophy.[67,68] It is more commonly seen on the left side (because the spermatic vein opens at a sharp angle into the left renal vein).[69] Dubin and Amelar's classification is a commonly used clinical grading assessment.[70] A large varicocele typically shows a "bag of worms" appearance on physical examination, and a smaller varicocele can be identified using the Valsalva maneuver.[70,71]

Renal Symptoms
PeVD caused by left renal vein obstruction (usually at the crossing of the aorta, NCS) can lead to renal venous hypertension and present with clinical symptoms of microhematuria or macrohematuria, proteinuria, or left flank pain[35] (see Fig. 3).

Extrapelvic Disorders
Lower extremity varicose veins of pelvic origin
PeVD is a common cause of lower extremity and vulvar varicose veins. It is caused by the transmission of pelvic venous hypertension from distal tributaries of the internal iliac vein into the veins of the lower extremity through the pelvic escape points (the inguinal, obturator, perineal, and gluteal)[7,15] (see Fig. 3). These atypical lower extremity varicose veins are usually not associated symptoms of CPP (potentially owing to decompression of pelvic venous pressure into the distal venous reservoir) or advanced lower extremity venous disease.[72,73] Pelvic reflux through the inguinal canal (escape point) can result in a bulging vein that can be misinterpreted as an indirect inguinal hernia. Obturator vein reflux through the obturator

point can result in varices of the medial proximal thigh. Internal pudendal reflux through the perineal escape point can result in varices of the posterior region of the vulva and proximal thigh. Inferior gluteal vein reflux through the gluteal escape point can result in varices of the posterior thigh and symptoms related to compression of the sciatic, common peroneal, and tibial nerves.[72] Therefore, patients presenting with nonsaphenous lower extremity varicosities must be examined for the involvement of the pelvis, upper thigh, and gluteal region to assess for PeVD and its involvement of lower extremity through the various pelvic escape points.

Venous claudication
Venous claudication is an exertional pain in the lower extremities, particularly in the thigh, buttock, or leg. It is usually not associated with a specific walking distance or muscle tenderness and is relieved by rest and leg elevation.[74–76] The most common cause of venous claudication is iliocaval venous obstruction.

Systemic Symptoms
Pulmonary emboli
MTS and NCS are characterized by mechanical compression of the left iliac and left renal veins, respectively. Chronic arterial pulsations and mechanical compression can lead to endothelial proliferation, vascular stenosis, and increased risk for the development of recurrent superficial vein and DVT.[44,50,77] DVT and acute pulmonary embolisms (PE) are clinical manifestations of venous thromboembolism. Clots from DVT can break off from vein walls and travel through the heart to the pulmonary arteries causing recurrent PE.

Chronic thromboembolic pulmonary hypertension

Chronic thromboembolic pulmonary hypertension is a progressive form of pulmonary hypertension caused by blood clots that do not dissolve in the lungs, causing a narrowing of the small artery and arterioles within the pulmonary vasculature.[78] The hallmark of this disorder is that it is relentlessly progressive, with the development of signs and symptoms of right heart failure and peripheral congestion, as well as decreased oxygenation. A history of blood clots in the lungs and elevated pulmonary pressures for at least 6 months after the diagnosis of PE is suggestive of chronic thromboembolic pulmonary hypertension.[78] The risk factors for chronic thromboembolic pulmonary hypertension coincide with those for pelvic venous obstruction, including hypercoagulability and prior leg DVT.[79]

Post-thrombotic (postphlebitic) syndrome

Post-thrombotic (postphlebitic) syndrome refers to signs and symptoms of chronic venous insufficiency that develop after a DVT.[80,81] It is caused by a combination of clot extension, damage to the venous valves, and the development of chronic regurgitation of the veins with venous hypertension, vascular engorgement, interstitial edema with pain, and chronic activation of the inflammatory cascade and sympathetic nervous system.[82,83] PTS can affect 23% to 60% of patients in the 2 years after a DVT of the leg.[84] Of those, 10% may go on to develop severe PTS involving venous ulcers.[84] Symptoms of leg pain, heaviness, itching or tingling, swelling, varicose veins, and skin discoloration are common. These symptoms worsen with walking and improve with leg elevation.[82,83]

Cardiovascular effects: cardiac preload reserve and heart failure: cardiovenous syndrome

Cardiac output increases by as much as 5-fold during exercise in the untrained man and by as much as 8-fold in the elite athlete. This increased venous return is a crucial part of the physiologic response to exercise. It is accomplished by the recruitment of preload reserve from the splanchnic compartment and extremities through the liver and central veins (iliac veins and vena cava). Therefore, obstruction in pelvic veins can potentially decrease venous return from the pelvis and lower extremities during exercise, leading to impaired preload reserve (cardiovenous syndrome), which may cause heart failure–like symptoms of exercise intolerance

(Fig. 5).[85] Although the preload reduced state (cardiovenous syndrome) might be similar in its presentation to heart failure with preserved ejection fraction, the central filling is low in preload reserve failure and high in heart failure with preserved ejection fraction.[85–87] Therefore, some authors have suggested that isolated preload reserve failure may be an underdiagnosed disorder. In a study by Oldham and colleagues[88] on patients with unexplained exertional dyspnea and evidence of reduced exercise performance, 18% of patients were noted to have isolated preload reserve limitation without evidence of heart failure with preserved ejection fraction.

In an extension of the cardiovenous syndrome, the inability to increase preload to the heart does not merely result in exercise-induced symptoms but in the extremes also likely results in resting symptoms. PeVD has been commonly described amongst patients with dysautonomia, such as postural tachycardia syndrome. Here, patients experience dizziness and fatigue with upright activities of daily living. Orthostatic intolerance is the cornerstone of this disease, marked by cerebral underperfusion. Dysautonomia patients (particularly postural tachycardia syndrome) exhibit a high prevalence of PeVD and the Ehlers–Danlos syndrome, which predisposes to soft tissue (and so also vascular tissue) abnormalities, likely predisposing abnormal venous pooling and vascular deformities as part of the PeVD described elsewhere in this article.[89]

Finally, the pain and interstitial edema associated with venous obstruction can be associated with activation of the adrenergic nervous system and inflammatory cascade.[90] This suggests that pelvic venous obstructions and interstitial or muscular edema may have a role in sympathetic nervous system activation, cardiac dysfunction, and chronic inflammation.[85]

DIAGNOSTIC APPROACH TO PELVIC VENOUS DISORDERS

PeVDs are generally considered only in patients with clinical evidence of persistently elevated lower extremity venous hydrostatic pressure not explained by cardiac or pericardial causes. However, defects of the pelvic veins may occur below the resting venous flow thresholds. Thus, the consideration of pelvic venous disease requires suspicion in patients who have a history of phlebitis or prior pregnancy resulting in pelvic venous valvular disruption and those patients who present with symptoms and syndromes that may reflect chronic pelvic congestion, recurrent DVT, pulmonary emboli (or their sequelae),

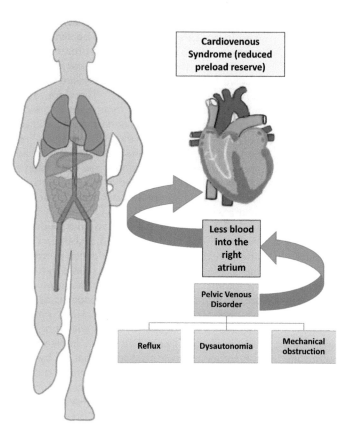

Fig. 5. An illustrative diagram showing cardiovenous syndrome (impaired preload reserve) owing to PeVD. PeVD is caused by mechanical venous obstruction, reflux (owing to incompetent valves), or dysautonomia (postural orthostatic tachycardia syndrome), leading to pooling of blood in venous reservoirs. This can potentially reduce the venous return from the pelvis and lower extremities during exercise, leading to impaired preload reserve (cardiovenous syndrome), which may cause exercise intolerance and heart failure-like symptoms.

resistant hypertension, or unexplained inflammation. Moreover, additional signs symptoms should add chronic pelvic venous diseases to the differential diagnosis. These symptoms include unexplained symmetric or asymmetrical gross leg edema or woody induration and skin breakdown often with superficial lower extremity varicosities, venous claudication defined as leg pain on exertion not associated with arterial insufficiency, chronic unexplained pelvic pain among women, engorgement of the pelvic venous plexus with gonadal and vulvar varicosities in association with CPP or specific obstetric and gynecologic presentations, unexplained hematuria and microhematuria with left renal vein engorgement or renal vein thrombosis, unexplained pulmonary emboli with or without pulmonary hypertension, and exercise intolerance owing to inadequate venous return to the heart, and even the resistance to hypertension medications.

A history and physical examination can help to narrow down the differential diagnosis toward PeVD; however, imaging is often needed to confirm the diagnosis and guide treatment. Traditionally, conventional venography is considered the gold standard for diagnosing PeVD.

However, it has been mostly replaced by less invasive modalities like ultrasound (US) examination, CT scans, and MRI. Cross-sectional imaging modalities such as CT scans and MRI can provide excellent anatomic details and good diagnostic accuracy and help to exclude alternative diagnoses such as endometriosis, uterine fibroids, and gynecologic malignancies. There are no standardized practice guidelines available on the use of diagnostic imaging for PeVD. Multiple factors, including the availability of imaging modality, local expertise, body habitus, and cost of imaging, can further complicate the individualized diagnostic approach.

The classical features associated with PeVD include pelvic varices, ovarian vein dilation, compression of the left common iliac and renal veins, pelvic origin extrapelvic varices, and lower extremity varices. On imaging, pelvic venous structures must be assessed for compression or luminal obstruction, asymmetrical flow, and presence of collaterals.

Conventional Venography

Venography is an invasive, catheter-based diagnostic modality. Although it is considered the gold standard for diagnosis of DVT, because of invasiveness, it is rarely performed.[91,92] It can also be performed to evaluate venous anatomy and collateral venous circulation before embolization.[93]

Ultrasound Examination

Real-time dynamic imaging, broad availability, lack of ionizing radiation, and the relatively lower cost make the US examination the ideal first-line imaging modality for evaluating PeVD and superficial venous disease. This practice is also recommended by Society for Vascular Surgery and the American Venous Forum.[94] Transabdominal, transvaginal or transperineal, and lower extremity US examination can allow a comprehensive assessment of the anatomy and underlying pathophysiology seen in different PeVDs.[95] It is important to perform the US examination in the supine, reclined, and standing positions and with Valsalva maneuver to see any potential obstruction and reflux by increasing hydrostatic pressure in the pelvic venous system. On the US examination, the veins are assessed for size, the direction of flow, and reflux (if reflux is not seen spontaneously, it can be elicited by the Valsalva maneuver).[95] The major limitations of US examinations include operator dependence, poor visualization of the deep pelvic venous structures (like ovarian vein reflux in the presence of bowel gas), and individuals with a large body habitus.[96]

In a study, Malgor and colleagues reported that the duplex US examination was able to demonstrate dilated left and right ovarian veins with a sensitivity of 100% and 90% and a specificity of 67% and 57%, respectively.[97] Positive predictive values for ovarian vein diameter of greater than 5 mm and of greater than 6 mm have been reported as 71.2% and 83.3%, respectively, for PeVD.[12] However, multiple studies have shown that ovarian vein size is an unreliable indicator of underlying PeVD and have suggested reflux (reversal of flow) as a better indicator of PeVD.[6,95,97] Steenbeek and colleagues[98] reported that ovarian vein reflux on transabdominal US examination had a sensitivity of 100% for the detection of PeVD. Another indicator is the presence of pelvic varicocele (dilated tortuous vein with a diameter of >4 mm), which has been shown to have high sensitivity (100%) and specificity (83%) for the detection of PeVD.[98]

Transvaginal US examinations can help to visualize structural changes in pelvic organs better than transabdominal US examinations. For instance, uterine (fibroids, tumors) and ovarian (polycystic changes, cysts) enlargement can cause venous compression. In a study, Whiteley and colleagues[99] noted 100% negative predictive value with no false positives and only 1 false negative in the patient population of 100 women. Multiple authors have suggested that venography should be replaced with the transvaginal US examination as the standard screening imaging modality for assessing PeVD.[95,99,100]

Computed Tomography Scans and MRI

CT scans and MRIs provide excellent anatomic details and can therefore help detect structural abnormalities and exclude nonvascular etiologies in evaluation for suspected PeVD. A CT scan can provide excellent visualization of venous anatomy, venous dilatation, and varices. However, on a CT scan, it is impossible to visualize the flow's direction (visualize the flow of contrast) if the gonadal veins and utero-ovarian arcade are completely filled.[12] This, combined with no ionizing radiation and excellent soft tissue contrast, make MRI a preferred modality over CT scans for the assessment of PeVD. An MRI allows evaluation of pelvic anatomy, including vascular structures as well as dynamic vascular flow.[12]

Three-plane high temporal resolution dynamic time-resolved T2-weighted MRI with multiplanar nonenhanced and contrast-enhanced multiplanar T1-weighted MRI and MR angiography are essential for the evaluation of PeVD.[101,102] One study comparing the diagnostic accuracy of conventional venography with MR angiography found an excellent agreement between the 2 modalities with sensitivity, specificity, and accuracy of 67% to 75%, 100%, and 79% to 84%, respectively.[101] One of the major limitations of MRI is that it cannot be used for follow-ups in patients with metallic coil insertion during embolization procedures.[103]

TREATMENT OF PELVIC VENOUS DISORDERS

It must be noted that, even though pelvic varicosities and compressive lesions are commonly seen on diagnostic imaging, they do not uniformly lead to disabling symptoms. For example, asymptomatic varicosities have been reported in 38% to 47% of women undergoing CT scans or MRI.[3] The treatment should be reserved for symptomatic patients.[104,105] Multiple treatment options are available for PeVD, including medical (hormonal therapies), surgical (hysterectomy, salpingo-oophorectomy, vein ligation), and endovascular options (transcatheter embolization and stenting). In addition, multiple pathologies can coexist, such as internal iliac vein incompetence and left renal vein compression. Therefore, for effective treatment of PeVD, an accurate diagnosis and understanding of the underlying pathophysiology of PeVD are crucial.

Medical Management

The medical treatment of PeVD is limited to conservative pain management. In patients with CPP (pelvic congestion syndrome), hormonal therapy targeted at ovarian suppression, with medroxyprogesterone acetate and gonadotropin-releasing hormone (goserelin) agonists can be attempted. However, these therapies are rarely used owing to their potential side effects (weight gain, menopausal symptoms, and osteoporosis) and low efficacy.[61,106,107] Nonsteroidal anti-inflammatory drugs can be used for symptomatic relief while undergoing evaluation before definitive treatment.[108] Various potential drugs for symptomatic relief remain under investigation.[109,110] For example, micronized purified flavonoid fraction, a venoactive drug, has shown encouraging results with a quicker resolution of symptoms compared with conventional therapy.[111,112]

Surgical Management

Surgical management is based on counteracting the mechanical factors involved in the pathogenesis of pelvic varicosities and obstruction. For example, hysterectomy with or without bilateral oophorectomy, resection, or ligation of the left ovarian vein (ovarian vein reflux) has been shown to relieve PeVD symptoms.[96,113,114] In PeVD with primary left renal vein compression (NCS), various procedures, namely, nephropexy, aortomesenteric transposition, renal autotransplantation, gonadal vein transposition, and left renal vein transposition, have been described.[3] For example, in NCS with left renal vein compression, a left ovarian vein transposition may lead to relief of NCS symptoms. In ovarian transposition to the IVC, the ovarian vein is mobilized and divided just above the pelvis, transposing it onto distal IVC or external iliac vein.[3]

Surgical management leads to longer hospital stays, higher mortality, high recurrence rates, and residual pain (in 20% and 33% of women after hysterectomy), as well as the potential risk of surgical complications (damage to nearby pelvic structures).[106,109,113,115,116] Therefore, a less invasive endovascular approach has largely replaced medical and surgical options for the management of PeVD.[113,116]

Endovascular Treatment

Endovascular is currently the preferred modality for the management of PeVD.[117,118] A number of percutaneous embolization (for vein insufficiency) and stent approaches (for vein stenosis) have been reported in the literature.

Endovascular treatment procedure

Endovascular procedures are typically done in an outpatient setting under sedation. First, under the US guidance, the right internal jugular vein or left femoral vein is canulated to perform diagnostic venography to visualize the pelvic venous structures (common iliac vein, external iliac vein, internal iliac vein, gonadal and left renal vein) to evaluate for reflux in internal iliac vein, and stenosis of the common iliac vein (MTS), stenosis of the left renal vein (NCS).[106,108] This step is followed by an embolization and/or stenting procedure based on the underlying pathophysiology. The clinical success of the procedure is measured by long-term symptomatic relief.

Embolization

Embolization is a relatively new modality, first described by Edwards and colleagues in 1993.[119] It is a safe and effective treatment modality for PeVD (caused by gonadal and pelvic vein insufficiency). The goal of transcatheter embolization is to occlude the pathologic refluxing veins, leading to a potential resolution of varicosities (through the resolution of increased hydrostatic pressure caused by refluxing vein).

Embolization agents

Various embolization agents, including coils, sclerosing agents, and glue, have been reported in the literature. Mechanical occlusion using metallic coils alone or combined with a sclerosing agent is one of the most commonly used techniques.[117,120] Coils usually comprise a metal core (stainless steel, platinum) and synthetic thrombogenic fibers from the body.[109] When introduced, the coil assumes the vessel's shape, leading to its mechanical occlusion and thrombosis.[117,120] Sclerosing agents (eg, sodium tetradecyl sulfate) come in various forms, including liquid, foam, and gelatin foam sponge.[121–123] Liquid sclerosing agents are often used behind the coil to ensure its stays in the right location and decrease the risk of extravasation. Foam agents can theoretically offer several advantages over liquid sclerosant, including larger surface contact with endothelium (leading to effective sclerosing) high viscosity (low risk of extravasation).[122,124] Glue agents (eg, a mixture of enbucrilate and iodized oil) can easily reflux into various affected collateral branches, leading to their effective thrombosis and occlusion. However, there is the risk of distal migration of glue fragments, including PE.

Outcome of pelvic venous embolization
Clinical success is measured by long-term symptomatic relief. Some of the reported complications of transcatheter embolization include, vein perforation (1%), transient pain (8%–100%), transient fever (12%), superficial thrombophlebitis at intervention site (9%), and coil migration (<2%).[125] Different vascular access sites and embolization agents have been used for transcatheter embolization in PeVD. However, there are no clinical studies comparing different embolization agents and procedure protocols. Therefore, the choice of approach and agent are based on individual operator preference and experience. In a literature review of various embolization studies using different agents, Meissner and colleagues[56] noted complete or partial symptom improvement in 68.2% to 100% of patients and a consistent reduction in visual analog pain scores after treatment. In a systemic review covering 14 studies and 828 women, Brown and colleagues[107] noted an improvement in clinical symptoms after endovascular treatment in 68.3% to 100% of patients. Some studies also suggest that embolization may treat infertility caused by venous congestion.[126,127]

Table 1
Rates of primary and secondary patency of stenting for nonthrombotic iliofemoral venous lesions

Author	Stent	N	F/U	Primary Patency (%)	Secondary Patency (%)	Complication
Attaran et al,[137] 2019	Wallstent	49	18 mo	97.8	100	2% occlusion
Dake et al,[138] 2021	Venovo	77	36 mo	97.1	-	-
De Wolf et al,[139] 2015	Sinus venous	35	12 mo	100	-	None
Hager et al,[140] 2013	Wallstent/ Protege	21	36 mo	91	91	9.4% stent thrombosis
Raju et al,[141] 2010	Wallstent	196	5 y	-	100	-
Gagne et al,[142] 2019	Wallstent	42	72 mo	97	100	-
Lichtenberg et al,[143] 2021	Venovo	29	2 y	95.5	100	1 occlusion
Rizivi et al,[144] 2018	Wallstent	210	2 y	97.9	-	1.5% in-stent thrombosis
George et al,[145] 2014	Niti (Taewong Medical, Seoul, Korea) Luminexx (Bard Peripheral Vascular)	35	15 mo	95	-	-
Liu et al,[146] 2014	Wallstent	32	1 y	96.9		3.1% DVT
Lou et al,[147] 2009	Luminexx (Bard, Murray Hill, NJ)	39	6 mo	92.6		

Patency was defined as uninterrupted venous patency (<50% diameter stenosis) without (primary) or with (secondary) a procedure or intervention directly performed on the target lesion.
Abbreviation: F/U, follow-up.

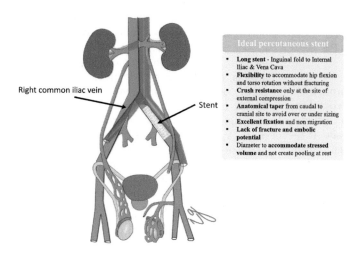

Right common iliac vein

Stent

Ideal percutaneous stent

- **Long stent** - Inguinal fold to Internal Iliac & Vena Cava
- **Flexibility** to accommodate hip flexion and torso rotation without fracturing
- **Crush resistance** only at the site of external compression
- **Anatomical taper** from caudal to cranial site to avoid over or under sizing
- **Excellent fixation** and non migration
- **Lack of fracture and embolic potential**
- Diameter to **accommodate stressed volume** and not create pooling at rest

Fig. 6. Ideal percutaneous venous stent.

Stenting for nonthrombotic iliac vein lesions
Deep venous stenting has been in practice for several decades to treat nonthrombotic iliac vein lesion and PTS. Although open surgery is possible, the relative safety and a higher reintervention rate seen in surgical treatment have steered therapy toward endovascular stenting.[128] Not surprisingly, the treatment of PTS results in lower patency rates than nonthrombotic iliac vein lesion owing to associated residual thrombus. Here we focus on nonthrombotic iliac vein lesion stenting results in PeVDs.

The treatment of nonthrombotic iliac vein lesion demands overcoming the compressive force of the common iliac artery, resistance to fracture and crushing, and fixation to the vessel without future concern for embolization. The pelvic venous anatomy is unique owing to the dispensability of the vasculature, vessel size mismatch owing to the possible need to stent from the IVC to the common femoral vein, and the flexion experienced in the pelvis and inguinal ligament. To accommodate these needs, most stents are made of laser-cut nitinol, except for the Wallstents (Boston Scientific-Schneider, Minneapolis, MN) made of woven elgiloy. There are several stents developed for venous stenting, but only 2 are approved by the US Food and Drug Administration; the Wallstents and Zilver Vena (Cook Medical, Bloomington, IN).[129]

Outcome of stenting and ideal stenting option. Nonthrombotic iliac vein lesion stenting is associated with low complication rates. A meta-analysis found a rate of 0.3% to 1.1% for significant bleeding and a 0.1% to 0.7% mortality rate. Primary patency rates vary from 91% to 100%. Still, it should be noted that most

data come from retrospective data, and there are few controlled trials characterizing the efficacy of venous stenting beyond 1 year (Table 1). The most common mechanisms of venous stenting failure include malposition of angulation of stent, acute DVT, stenosis in native iliac vein proximal or distal to the original lesion, in-stent restenosis, and impairment of flow from the contralateral vessel from the previously placed stent.[130] Stent migration or embolization was not reported in the published cases series, but several episodes of stent embolization have occurred, prompting product recalls from 2 different manufacturers.[131–133] Stent fracture is seldom discussed in venous stenting literature, likely owing to variability in surveillance in follow-up.[134] To create an ideal percutaneous stenting solution, the challenges of the current stent design causing malpositioning, thrombus formation, restenosis, migration, or embolization need to be addressed (Fig. 6).

Follow-up
A follow-up examination is recommended for the reassessment of chronic symptoms in 3 to 6 months. If the patient has persistent symptoms, imaging evaluation and percutaneous embolization or restenting of the venous pathway may be needed.[135,136]

SUMMARY

PeVD can present with a wide spectrum of clinical features. Understanding the underlying pathophysiological mechanism of these disorders is crucial for the appropriate diagnosis and treatment of these patients. There are no standardized guidelines, and, therefore, for optimal outcomes, the diagnostic and therapeutic approach must be individually tailored. Although multiple treatment options are available, endovascular is becoming the mainstay of management of PeVD patients owing to a higher success rate with a lower risk of complications. However, further studies are needed to investigate the long-term outcomes.

CLINICS CARE POINTS

- Understanding underlying pathophysiology, including pelvic venous anatomy (normal and abnormal variants), drainage pathway of interconnected venous reservoirs, and various risk factors, can help optimize diagnosis and treatment.

- Asymptomatic pelvic venous varicosities are often seen as an incidental finding on CT scans or MRI. Treatment should only be reserved for symptomatic patients.

- In patients presenting with CPP, imaging (CT scans and MRI) can help to visualize the pelvic vascular and visceral structures to confirm PeVD and rule out other potential (gynecologic, gastrointestinal, and urologic) causes of CPP.

- Although percutaneous interventions have shown encouraging treatment results, further studies are needed to assess their long-term outcomes.

DISCLOSURE

Dr Fudim was supported by the National Heart, Lung, and Blood Institute (NHLBI) (K23HL151744), the American Heart Association (20IPA35310955), Mario Family Award, Duke Chair's Award, Translating Duke Health Award, Bayer, Bodyport, BTG Specialty Pharmaceuticals and Verily. He receives consulting fees from Abbott, Alleviant, Audicor, AxonTherapies, Bayer, Bodyguide, Bodyport, Boston Scientific, CVRx, Daxor, Deerfield Catalyst, Edwards Life-Sciences, Feldschuh Foundation, Fire1, Gradient, Intershunt, NXT Biomedical, Pharmacosmos, PreHealth, Shifamed, Splendo, Vironix, Viscardia, Zoll. Dr. Paul A. Sabotka is founder of V-Flow inc.

REFERENCES

1. Lazarashvili Z, Antignani PL, Monedero JL. Pelvic congestion syndrome: prevalence and quality of life. Phlebolymphology 2016;23(3):123–6.

2. Belenky A, Bartal G, Atar E, et al. Ovarian varices in healthy female kidney donors: incidence, morbidity, and clinical outcome. AJR Am J Roentgenol 2002;179(3):625–7.

3. Meissner MH, Gloviczki P. Pelvic venous disorders, in Atlas of endovascular venous surgery. Elsevier (Amsterdam): Pelvic Venous Disorders; 2019. p. 567–99.

4. Khilnani NM, Meissner MH, Learman LA, et al. Research priorities in pelvic venous disorders in women: recommendations from a multidisciplinary research consensus panel. J Vasc Interv Radiol 2019;30(6):781–9.

5. Eklöf B, Rutherford RB, Bergan JJ, et al. Revision of the CEAP classification for chronic venous disorders: consensus statement. J Vasc Surg 2004; 40(6):1248–52.

6. Borghi C, Dell'Atti L. Pelvic congestion syndrome: the current state of the literature. Arch Gynecol Obstet 2016;293(2):291–301.

7. Meissner MH, Khilnani NM, Labropoulos N, et al. The symptoms-varices-pathophysiology classification of pelvic venous disorders: a report of the American Vein & Lymphatic Society International Working Group on Pelvic Venous Disorders. Phlebology 2021;36(5):342–60.

8. Basile A, Castiglione D. The Symptoms-Varices-Pathophysiology (SVP) Classification of Pelvic Venous Disorders": a new tool to assess the complex scenario of chronic venous diseases. Cardiovasc Intervent Radiol 2021;44(8):1298–9.

9. Jeppson PC, Balgobin S, Washington BB, et al. Recommended standardized terminology of the anterior female pelvis based on a structured medical literature review. Am J Obstet Gynecol 2018; 219(1):26–39.

10. Balgobin S, Jeppson PC, Wheeler T, et al. Standardized terminology of apical structures in the female pelvis based on a structured medical literature review. Am J Obstet Gynecol 2020;222(3): 204–18.

11. Beckett D, Dos Santos SJ, Dabbs EB, et al. Anatomical abnormalities of the pelvic venous system and their implications for endovascular management of pelvic venous reflux. Phlebology 2018;33(8):567–74.

12. Bookwalter CA, VanBuren WM, Neisen MJ, et al. Imaging appearance and nonsurgical management of pelvic venous congestion syndrome. Radiographics 2019;39(2):596–608.

13. Phillips D, Deipolyi AR, Hesketh RL, et al. Pelvic congestion syndrome: etiology of pain, diagnosis, and clinical management. J Vasc Interv Radiol 2014;25(5):725–33.

14. Heinz A, Brenner F. Valves of the gonadal veins. Phlebologie 2010;39(06):317–24.

15. Lemasle P, Greiner M. Duplex ultrasound investigation in pelvic congestion syndrome: technique and results. Phlebolymphology 2017;24(2):79–87.

16. Kachlik D, Pechacek V, Musil V, et al. The venous system of the pelvis: new nomenclature. Phlebology 2010;25(4):162–73.

17. Whiteley MS, Dabbs EB, Davis EL, et al. Response to "Commentary on pelvic venous reflux in males with varicose veins and recurrent varicose veins". Phlebology 2019;34(1):70–1.

18. Doganci S. Poorly understood pelvic venous disorders require a multidisciplinary approach. Phlebologie 2021;50(04):279–82.

19. Christenson BM, Gipson MG, Smith MT. Pelvic vascular malformations. In: Seminars in interventional radiology. New York: Thieme Medical Publishers; 2013. p. 364–71.

20. Winer AG, Chakiryan NH, Mooney RP, et al. Secondary pelvic congestion syndrome: description and radiographic diagnosis. Can J Urol 2014;21(4):7365–8.

21. Menezes T, Haider EA, Al-Douri F, et al. Pelvic congestion syndrome due to agenesis of the infrarenal inferior vena cava. Radiol Case Rep 2019;14(1):36–40.

22. Singh SN, Bhatt TC. Inferior vena cava agenesis: a rare cause of pelvic congestion syndrome. J Clin Diagn Res 2017;11(3):TD06.

23. Sharma M, Rameshbabu CS. Collateral pathways in portal hypertension. J Clin Exp Hepatol 2012;2(4):338–52.

24. Perry CP. Current concepts of pelvic congestion and chronic pelvic pain. JSLS 2001;5(2):105, 10.

25. Marques A, Peralta M, Naia A, et al. Prevalence of adult overweight and obesity in 20 European countries, 2014. Eur J Public Health 2018;28(2):295–300.

26. Reilly JJ, El-Hamdouchi A, Diouf A, et al. Determining the worldwide prevalence of obesity. Lancet 2018;391(10132):1773–4.

27. Ward ZJ, Bleich SN, Cradock AL, et al. Projected U.S. State-Level Prevalence of Adult Obesity and Severe Obesity. N Engl J Med 2019;381(25):2440–50.

28. Van Rij AM, De Alwis CS, Jiang P, et al. Obesity and impaired venous function. Eur J Vasc Endovasc Surg 2008;35(6):739–44.

29. Varela JE, Hinojosa M, Nguyen N. Correlations between intra-abdominal pressure and obesity-related co-morbidities. Surg Obes Relat Dis 2009;5(5):524–8.

30. De Keulenaer BL, De Waele JJ, Powell B, et al. What is normal intra-abdominal pressure and how is it affected by positioning, body mass and positive end-expiratory pressure? Intensive Care Med 2009;35(6):969–76.

31. Brice G, Mansour S, Bell R, et al. Analysis of the phenotypic abnormalities in lymphoedema-distichiasis syndrome in 74 patients with FOXC2 mutations or linkage to 16q24. J Med Genet 2002;39(7):478–83.

32. Asciutto G, Mumme A, Asciutto KC, et al. Oestradiol levels in varicose vein blood of patients with and without pelvic vein incompetence (PVI): diagnostic implications. Eur J Vasc Endovasc Surg 2010;40(1):117–21.

33. Raffetto JD, Khalil RA. Mechanisms of varicose vein formation: valve dysfunction and wall dilation. Phlebology 2008;23(2):85–98.

34. Sichlau MJ, Yao JS, Vogelzang RL. Transcatheter embolotherapy for the treatment of pelvic congestion syndrome. Obstet Gynecol 1994;83(5 Pt 2):892–6.

35. Kurklinsky AK, Rooke TW. Nutcracker phenomenon and nutcracker syndrome. Elsevier Rochester: Mayo clinic proceedings; 2010:85. p. 552–559.

36. De Schepper A. Nutcracker" phenomenon of the renal vein and venous pathology of the left kidney. J Belge Radiol 1972;55(5):507–11.

37. Kahn PC. Selective venography of the branches. Venography of the inferior vena cava and its branches. Huntington (WA): Krieger; 1973. p. 154–224.

38. Karaman B, Koplay M, Ozturk E, et al. Retroaortic left renal vein: multidetector computed tomography angiography findings and its clinical importance. Acta Radiol 2007;48(3):355–60.

39. Fong JK, Poh AC, Tan AG, et al. Imaging findings and clinical features of abdominal vascular compression syndromes. AJR Am J Roentgenol 2014;203(1):29–36.

40. Polguj M, Topol M, Majos A. An unusual case of left venous renal entrapment syndrome: a new type of nutcracker phenomenon? Surg Radiol Anat 2013;35(3):263–7.

41. Zhang H, Li M, Jin W, et al. The left renal entrapment syndrome: diagnosis and treatment. Ann Vasc Surg 2007;21(2):198–203.

42. Holdstock JM, Dos Santos SJ, Harrison CC, et al. Haemorrhoids are associated with internal iliac vein reflux in up to one-third of women presenting with varicose veins associated with pelvic vein reflux. Phlebology 2015;30(2):133–9.

43. Grimm LJ, Engstrom BI, Nelson RC, et al. Incidental detection of nutcracker phenomenon on multidetector CT in an asymptomatic population: prevalence and associated findings. J Comput Assist Tomogr 2013;37(3):415–8.

44. Butros SR, Liu R, Oliveira GR, et al. Venous compression syndromes: clinical features, imaging findings and management. Br J Radiol 2013;86(1030):20130284.

45. Fretz V, Binkert CA. Compression of the inferior vena cava by the right iliac artery: a rare variant of May–Thurner syndrome. Cardiovasc Intervent Radiol 2010;33(5):1060–3.

46. Burke RM, Rayan SS, Kasirajan K, et al. Unusual case of right-sided May-Thurner syndrome and review of its management. Vascular 2006;14(1):47–50.

47. Ibrahim W, Al Safran Z, Hasan H, et al. Endovascular management of May-Thurner syndrome. Ann Vasc Dis 2012;5(2):217–21.

48. Murphy EH, Davis CM, Journeycake JM, et al. Symptomatic iliofemoral DVT after onset of oral contraceptive use in women with previously undiagnosed May-Thurner Syndrome. J Vasc Surg 2009;49(3):697–703.

49. Cockett FB, Thomas ML. The iliac compression syndrome. Br J Surg 1965;52(10):816–21.

50. May R, Thurner J. The cause of the predominantly sinistral occurrence of thrombosis of the pelvic veins. Angiology 1957;8(5):419–27.

51. Birn J, Vedantham S. May–Thurner syndrome and other obstructive iliac vein lesions: meaning, myth, and mystery. Vasc Med 2015;20(1):74–83.

52. Knuttinen MG, Naidu S, Oklu R, et al. May-Thurner: diagnosis and endovascular management. Cardiovasc Diagn Ther 2017;7(Suppl 3):S159.

53. Meissner MH, Gloviczki P, Comerota AJ, et al. Early thrombus removal strategies for acute deep venous thrombosis: clinical practice guidelines of the Society for Vascular Surgery and the American Venous Forum. J Vasc Surg 2012;55(5):1449–62.

54. Khilnani NM, Winokur RS, Scherer KL, et al. Clinical presentation and evaluation of pelvic venous disorders in women. Tech Vasc Interv Radiol 2021;24(1):100730.

55. Greiner M, Dadon M, Lemasle P, et al. How does the pathophysiology influence the treatment of pelvic congestion syndrome and is the result long-lasting? Phlebology 2012;27 Suppl 1(1_suppl):58–64.

56. Meissner MH, Gibson K. Clinical outcome after treatment of pelvic congestion syndrome: sense and nonsense. Phlebology 2015;30(1_suppl):73–80.

57. Eklof B, Perrin M, Delis KT, et al. Updated terminology of chronic venous disorders: the VEIN-TERM transatlantic interdisciplinary consensus document. J Vasc Surg 2009;49(2):498–501.

58. Sulakvelidze L, Tran M, Kennedy R, et al. Presentation patterns in women with pelvic venous disorders differ based on age of presentation. Phlebology 2021;36(2):135–44.

59. Okaro E, Condous G, Khalid A, et al. The use of ultrasound-based 'soft markers' for the prediction of pelvic pathology in women with chronic pelvic pain—can we reduce the need for laparoscopy? BJOG 2006;113(3):251–6.

60. Zondervan KT, Yudkin PL, Vessey MP, et al. Chronic pelvic pain in the community—symptoms, investigations, and diagnoses. Am J Obstet Gynecol 2001;184(6):1149–55.

61. Soysal ME, Soysal S, Vicdan K, et al. A randomized controlled trial of goserelin and medroxyprogesterone acetate in the treatment of pelvic congestion. Hum Reprod 2001;16(5):931–9.

62. Hobbs JT. The pelvic congestion syndrome. Br J Hosp Med 1990;43(3):200–6.

63. Herrera-Betancourt AL, Villegas-Echeverri JD, López-Jaramillo JD, et al. Sensitivity and specificity of clinical findings for the diagnosis of pelvic congestion syndrome in women with chronic pelvic pain. Phlebology 2018;33(5):303–8.

64. Potts JM. Chronic pelvic pain syndrome: a non-prostatocentric perspective. World J Urol 2003;21(2):54–6.

65. Rana N, Drake MJ, Rinko R, et al. The fundamentals of chronic pelvic pain assessment, based on international continence society recommendations. Neurourol Urodyn 2018;37(S6):S32–8.

66. Paick S, Choi WS. Varicocele and testicular pain: a review. World J Mens Health 2019;37(1):4–11.

67. Agarwal A, Makker K, Sharma R. Clinical relevance of oxidative stress in male factor infertility: an update. Am J Reprod Immunol 2008;59(1):2–11.

68. Eisenberg ML, Lipshultz LI. Varicocele-induced infertility: newer insights into its pathophysiology. Indian J Urol 2011;27(1):58–64.

69. Stahl P, Schlegel PN. Standardization and documentation of varicocele evaluation. Curr Opin Urol 2011;21(6):500–5.

70. Dubin L, Amelar RD. Varicocele size and results of varicocelectomy in selected subfertile men with varicocele. Fertil Steril 1970;21(8):606–9.

71. Brahmbhatt A, Macher J, Shetty AN, et al. Sonographic evaluation of pelvic venous disorders. Ultrasound Q 2021;37(3):219–28.

72. Malgor RD, Labropoulos N. Pattern and types of non-saphenous vein reflux. Phlebology 2013;28 Suppl 1(1_suppl):51–4.

73. Gibson K, Minjarez R, Ferris B, et al. Clinical presentation of women with pelvic source varicose veins in the perineum as a first step in the development of a disease-specific patient assessment tool. J Vasc Surg Venous Lymphat Disord 2017;5(4):493–9.

74. Gloviczki P, Cho J. Surgical treatment of chronic occlusions of the iliac veins and the inferior vena cava. Vasc Surg 2005;2:2303–20.

75. Perrin M, Eklof B, VAN Rij A, et al. Venous symptoms: the SYM Vein Consensus statement developed under the auspices of the European Venous Forum. Int Angiol 2016;35(4):374–98.

76. Meissner MH, Eklof B, Smith PC, et al. Secondary chronic venous disorders. J Vasc Surg 2007;46 Suppl S(6):68S–83S.

77. Esposito A, Charisis N, Kantarovsky A, et al. A comprehensive review of the pathophysiology and clinical importance of iliac vein obstruction. Eur J Vasc Endovasc Surg 2020;60(1):118–25.

78. Hoeper MM, Mayer E, Simonneau G, et al. Chronic thromboembolic pulmonary hypertension. Circulation 2006;113(16):2011–20.

79. Al-Otaibi M, Vaidy A, Vaidya A, et al. May-Thurner anatomy in patients with chronic thromboembolic pulmonary hypertension: an important clinical association. JACC Cardiovasc Interv 2021;14(17):1940–6.

80. Grosse SD, Nelson RE, Nyarko KA, et al. The economic burden of incident venous thromboembolism in the United States: a review of estimated attributable healthcare costs. Thromb Res 2016;137:3–10.

81. Kahn SR, Partsch H, Vedantham S, et al. Definition of post-thrombotic syndrome of the leg for use in clinical investigations: a recommendation for standardization. J Thromb Haemost 2009;7(5):879–83.

82. Bergan JJ, Schmid-Schönbein GW, Smith PD, et al. Chronic venous disease. N Engl J Med 2006;355(5):488–98.

83. Franzeck UK, Schalch I, Jäger KA, et al. Prospective 12-year follow-up study of clinical and hemodynamic sequelae after deep vein thrombosis in low-risk patients (Zürich study). Circulation 1996;93(1):74–9.

84. Prandoni P, Kahn SR. Post-thrombotic syndrome: prevalence, prognostication and need for progress. Br J Haematol 2009;145(3):286–95.

85. Fudim M, Sobotka PA, Dunlap ME. Extracardiac abnormalities of preload reserve: mechanisms underlying exercise limitation in heart failure with preserved ejection fraction, autonomic dysfunction, and liver disease. Circ Heart Fail 2021;14(1):e007308.

86. Pfeffer MA, Shah AM, Borlaug BA. Heart failure with preserved ejection fraction in perspective. Circ Res 2019;124(11):1598–617.

87. Rao VN, Kelsey MD, Blazing MA, et al. Unexplained dyspnea on exertion: the difference the right test can make. Circ Heart Fail; 2022.

88. Oldham WM, Lewis GD, Opotowsky AR, et al. Unexplained exertional dyspnea caused by low ventricular filling pressures: results from clinical invasive cardiopulmonary exercise testing. Pulm Circ 2016;6(1):55–62.

89. Roma M, Marden CL, De Wandele I, et al. Postural tachycardia syndrome and other forms of orthostatic intolerance in Ehlers-Danlos syndrome. Auton Neurosci 2018;215:89–96.

90. McClain J, Hardy C, Enders B, et al. Limb congestion and sympathoexcitation during exercise.

Implications for congestive heart failure. J Clin Invest 1993;92:2353–9.

91. Ganeshan A, Upponi S, Hon LQ, et al. Chronic pelvic pain due to pelvic congestion syndrome: the role of diagnostic and interventional radiology. Cardiovasc Intervent Radiol 2007;30(6):1105–11.

92. Bates SM, Jaeschke R, Stevens SM, et al. Diagnosis of DVT: antithrombotic therapy and prevention of thrombosis, 9th ed: American College of Chest Physicians Evidence-Based Clinical Practice Guidelines. Chest 2012;141(2 Suppl):e351S–418S.

93. Marcelin C, Izaaryene J, Castelli M, et al. Embolization of ovarian vein for pelvic congestion syndrome with ethylene vinyl alcohol copolymer (Onyx®). Diagn Interv Imaging 2017;98(12):843–8.

94. Gloviczki P, Comerota AJ, Dalsing MC, et al. Society for Vascular Surgery; American Venous Forum. The care of patients with varicose veins and associated chronic venous diseases: clinical practice guidelines of the Society for Vascular Surgery and the American Venous Forum. J Vasc Surg 2011;53:2S–48S.

95. Labropoulos N, Jasinski PT, Adrahtas D, et al. A standardized ultrasound approach to pelvic congestion syndrome. Phlebology 2017;32(9):608–19.

96. Stones RW. Pelvic vascular congestion—half a century later. Clin Obstet Gynecol 2003;46(4):831–6.

97. Malgor RD, Adrahtas D, Spentzouris G, et al. The role of duplex ultrasound in the workup of pelvic congestion syndrome. J Vasc Surg Venous Lymphat Disord 2014;2(1):34–8.

98. Steenbeek MP, van der Vleuten CJM, Schultze Kool LJ, et al. Noninvasive diagnostic tools for pelvic congestion syndrome: a systematic review. Acta Obstet Gynecol Scand 2018;97(7):776–86.

99. Whiteley MS, Dos Santos SJ, Harrison CC, et al. Transvaginal duplex ultrasonography appears to be the gold standard investigation for the haemodynamic evaluation of pelvic venous reflux in the ovarian and internal iliac veins in women. Phlebology 2015;30(10):706–13.

100. Hansrani V, Dhorat Z, McCollum CN. Diagnosing of pelvic vein incompetence using minimally invasive ultrasound techniques. Vascular 2017;25(3):253–9.

101. Yang DM, Kim HC, Nam DH, et al. Time-resolved MR angiography for detecting and grading ovarian venous reflux: comparison with conventional venography. Br J Radiol 2012;85(1014):e117-22.

102. Pandey T, Shaikh R, Viswamitra S, et al. Use of time resolved magnetic resonance imaging in the diagnosis of pelvic congestion syndrome. J Magn Reson Imaging 2010;32(3):700–4.

103. Arnoldussen CW, de Wolf MA, Wittens CH. Diagnostic imaging of pelvic congestive syndrome. Phlebology 2015;30(1_suppl):67–72.

104. White JM, Comerota AJ. Venous compression syndromes. Vasc Endovascular Surg 2017;51(3):155–68.

105. Kahn SR, Comerota AJ, Cushman M, et al. The postthrombotic syndrome: evidence-based prevention, diagnosis, and treatment strategies: a scientific statement from the American Heart Association. Circulation 2014;130(18):1636–61.

106. Ignacio EA, Dua R, Sarin S, et al. Pelvic congestion syndrome: diagnosis and treatment. Semin Intervent Radiol 2008;25:361–8.

107. Brown CL, Rizer M, Alexander R, et al. Pelvic Congestion Syndrome: Systematic Review of Treatment Success. Semin Intervent Radiol 2018;35:35–40.

108. Mahmoud O, Vikatmaa P, Aho P, et al. Efficacy of endovascular treatment for pelvic congestion syndrome. J Vasc Surg Venous Lymphat Disord 2016;4(3):355–70.

109. Knuttinen MG, Xie K, Jani A, et al. Pelvic venous insufficiency: imaging diagnosis, treatment approaches, and therapeutic issues. AJR Am J Roentgenol 2015;204(2):448–58.

110. Shokeir T, Amr M, Abdelshaheed M. The efficacy of Implanon for the treatment of chronic pelvic pain associated with pelvic congestion: 1-year randomized controlled pilot study. Arch Gynecol Obstet 2009;280(3):437–43.

111. Sahin A, Kutluhan MA, Yildirim C, et al. Results of purified micronized flavonoid fraction in the treatment of categorized type III chronic pelvic pain syndrome: a randomized controlled trial. Aging Male 2020;23(5):1103–8.

112. Gavrilov SG, Karalkin AV, Moskalenko YP, et al. Efficacy of two micronized purified flavonoid fraction dosing regimens in the pelvic venous pain relie. Int Angiol 2021;40:180–6.

113. Salani R, Backes FJ, Fung MF, et al. Posttreatment surveillance and diagnosis of recurrence in women with gynecologic malignancies: Society of Gynecologic Oncologists recommendations. Am J Obstet Gynecol 2011;204(6):466–78.

114. Takeuchi K, Mochizuki M, Kitagaki S. Laparoscopic varicocele ligation for pelvic congestion syndrome. Int J Gynaecol Obstet 1996;55(2):177–8.

115. Almeida GR, Silvinato A, Simões RS, et al. Pelvic congestion syndrome - treatment with pelvic varicose veins embolization. Rev Assoc Med Bras (1992) 2019;65:518–23.

116. Corrêa MP, Bianchini L, Saleh JN, et al. Pelvic congestion syndrome and embolization of pelvic varicose veins. J Vasc Bras 2019;18:e20190061

117. Venbrux AC, Chang AH, Kim HS, et al. Pelvic congestion syndrome (pelvic venous incompetence): impact of ovarian and internal iliac vein embolotherapy on menstrual cycle and chronic pelvic pain. J Vasc Interv Radiol 2002;13(2):171–8.

118. Laborda A, Medrano J, de Blas I, et al. Endovascular treatment of pelvic congestion syndrome: visual analog scale (VAS) long-term follow-up clinical evaluation in 202 patients. Cardiovasc Intervent Radiol 2013;36(4):1006–14.

119. Edwards RD, Robertson IR, MacLean AB, et al. Case report: pelvic pain syndrome–successful treatment of a case by ovarian vein embolization. Clin Radiol 1993;47(6):429–31.

120. Tu FF, Hahn D, Steege JF. Pelvic congestion syndrome-associated pelvic pain: a systematic review of diagnosis and management. Obstet Gynecol Surv 2010;65(5):332–40.

121. Kwon SH, Oh JH, Ko KR, et al. Transcatheter ovarian vein embolization using coils for the treatment of pelvic congestion syndrome. Cardiovasc Intervent Radiol 2007;30(4):655–61.

122. Tessari L, Cavezzi A, Frullini A. Preliminary experience with a new sclerosing foam in the treatment of varicose veins. Dermatol Surg 2001;27(1):58–60.

123. Meneses L, Fava M, Diaz P, et al. Embolization of incompetent pelvic veins for the treatment of recurrent varicose veins in lower limbs and pelvic congestion syndrome. Cardiovasc Intervent Radiol 2013;36(1):128–32.

124. Gandini R, Chiocchi M, Konda D, et al. Transcatheter foam sclerotherapy of symptomatic female varicocele with sodium-tetradecyl-sulfate foam. Cardiovasc Intervent Radiol 2008;31(4):778–84.

125. Whiteley MS, Lewis-Shiell C, Bishop SI, et al. Pelvic vein embolisation of gonadal and internal iliac veins can be performed safely and with good technical results in an ambulatory vein clinic, under local anaesthetic alone - Results from two years' experience. Phlebology 2018;33(8):575–9.

126. Santoshi RKN, Lakhanpal S, Satwah V, et al. Iliac vein stenosis is an underdiagnosed cause of pelvic venous insufficiency. J Vasc Surg Venous Lymphat Disord 2018;6(2):202–11.

127. Tarazov P, Prozorovskij K, Rumiantseva S. Pregnancy after embolization of an ovarian varicocele associated with infertility: report of two cases. Diagn Interv Radiol 2011;17(2):174, 6.

128. Galanakis N, Kontopodis N, Kehagias E, et al. Direct Iliac Vein Stenting in Phlegmasia Cerulea Dolens Caused by May–Thurner Syndrome. Vasc Specialist Int 2021;37:37.

129. Dabir D, Feisst A, Thomas D, et al. Physical properties of venous stents: an experimental comparison. Cardiovasc Intervent Radiol 2018;41(6):942–50.

130. Aboubakr A, Chait J, Lurie J, et al. Secondary interventions after iliac vein stenting for chronic

proximal venous outflow obstruction. J Vasc Surg Venous Lymphat Disord 2019;7(5):670–6.

131. Caton MT Jr, Brown JM, Steigner ML. Iliac Stent Migration to the Right Ventricular Outflow Tract. Circ Cardiovasc Imaging 2018;11(12):e008520.

132. Orellana-Barrios M, Patel N, Arvandi A, et al. Venous stent migration into right ventricle. Cureus 2017;9(8):e1583.

133. Chick JFB, Gemmete JJ, Hage AN, et al. Stent placement across the renal vein inflow in patients undergoing venous reconstruction preserves renal function and renal vein patency: experience in 93 patients. J Endovasc Ther 2019;26(2):258–64.

134. Machado H, Sousa J, Mansilha A. The impact of venous stenting across the inguinal ligament on primary patency: a systematic review. Int Angiol 2021;40(4):270–6.

135. Tuite DJ, Kessel DO, Nicholson AA, et al. Initial clinical experience using the Amplatzer vascular plug. Cardiovasc Intervent Radiol 2007;30(4):650–4.

136. Basile A, Marletta G, Tsetis D, et al. The Amplatzer vascular plug also for ovarian vein embolization. Cardiovasc Intervent Radiol 2008;31(2):446–7.

137. Attaran RR, Ozdemir D, Lin IH, et al. Evaluation of anticoagulant and antiplatelet therapy after iliocaval stenting: factors associated with stent occlusion. J Vasc Surg Venous Lymphat Disord 2019;7(4):527–34.

138. Dake MD, O'Sullivan G, Shammas NW, et al. Three-year results from the venovo venous stent study for the treatment of iliac and femoral vein obstruction. Cardiovasc Intervent Radiol 2021;44(12):1918–29.

139. De Wolf MA, de Graaf R, Kurstjens RL, et al. Short-term clinical experience with a dedicated venous nitinol stent: initial results with the sinus-venous stent. Eur J Vasc Endovasc Surg 2015;50(4):518–26.

140. Hager ES, Yuo T, Tahara R, et al. Outcomes of endovascular intervention for May-Thurner syndrome. J Vasc Surg Venous Lymphat Disord 2013;1(3):270–5.

141. Raju S, Darcey R, Neglén P. Unexpected major role for venous stenting in deep reflux disease. J Vasc Surg 2010;51(2):401–8.

142. Gagne PJ, Gagne N, Kucher T, et al. Long-term clinical outcomes and technical factors with the Wallstent for treatment of chronic iliofemoral venous obstruction. J Vasc Surg Venous Lymphat Disord 2019;7(1):45–55.

143. Lichtenberg M, Zeller T, Gaines P, et al. MIMICS-3D investigators. BioMimics 3D vascular stent system for femoropopliteal interventions. Vasa 2022;51:5–12.

144. Rizvi SA, Ascher E, Hingorani A, et al. Stent patency in patients with advanced chronic venous disease and nonthrombotic iliac vein lesions. J Vasc Surg Venous Lymphat Disord 2018;6(4):457–63.

145. George R, Verma H, Ram B, et al. Re. "The effect of deep venous stenting on healing of lower limb venous ulcers". Eur J Vasc Endovasc Surg 2014;48(3):711, 336.

146. Liu Z, Gao N, Shen L, et al. Endovascular treatment for symptomatic iliac vein compression syndrome: a prospective consecutive series of 48 patients. Ann Vasc Surg 2014;28(3):695–704.

147. Lou WS, Gu JP, He X, et al. Endovascular treatment for iliac vein compression syndrome: a comparison between the presence and absence of secondary thrombosis. Korean J Radiol 2009;10(2):135–43.

Management Principles for the Cardiac Catheterization Laboratory During the Severe Acute Respiratory Syndrome Coronavirus-2 (SARS-CoV-2) Pandemic

Keshav R. Nayak, MD, FACC, FSCAI[a],*,
Ryan C. Maves, MD, FCCM, FCCP, FIDSA[b,c],
Timothy D. Henry, MD, FACC, MSCAI[d,e]

KEYWORDS

- Cardiac catheterization laboratory • Coronavirus • Pandemic • COVID-19 vaccination status
- COVID-19 positive status • PPE • Infection control • Quality control

KEY POINTS

- The severe acute respiratory syndrome coronavirus-2 (SARS-CoV-2) is a highly contagious pathogen. The resulting illness, 2019 coronavirus disease (COVID-19), has significant morbidity and mortality and has a direct impact on cardiac catheterization laboratory (CCL) operations. The CCL needs formal preparedness protocols for safe, effective, and timely operations. There is a dire need for consensus evidence-based guidance and guidelines from international heart associations.
- CCL teams are frontline workers, similar to the emergency room and critical care teams. They directly care for patients with cardiovascular emergencies, including but not limited to ST-segment elevation MI (STEMI), in suspected or confirmed infected patients.
- Infection control Principles center on 3 levels of hierarchical controls: (a) protection of the health care worker with personal protective equipment (PPE), (b) administrative (staff training, restriction of nonessential personnel with an optimized staffing matrix), and (c) environmental/engineering controls (social distancing, isolation of personnel from the infectious hazard).
- All CCL staff in direct contact with potentially infectious patients should be provided with N95 respirators, whole face shields or protective eyewear, disposable caps, shoe covers, sterile gowns, and surgical gloves. Powered air-purifying respirators (PAPRs) are an acceptable alternative for staff who cannot wear N95 respirators.
- CCL readiness and sustainable continuation of operations should be the goal during global pandemics to provide emergency care for at-risk cardiac patients who are the most vulnerable to poor outcomes. Delays in nonemergent procedures may be necessary during major pandemic surges but cannot be deferred indefinitely.

[a] Department of Cardiology, Scripps Mercy Hospital San Diego, 4077 Fifth Avenue, San Diego, CA 92103, USA; [b] Department of Internal Medicine, Wake Forest School of Medicine, 300 Medical Center Boulevard, Winston-Salem, NC 27157, USA; [c] Department of Anesthesiology, Wake Forest School of Medicine, 300 Medical Center Boulevard, Winston-Salem, NC 27157, USA; [d] The Carl and Edyth Lindner Center for Research and Education, 2123 Auburn Avenue Ste 424, Cincinnati, OH 45219, USA; [e] The Christ Hospital, 2139 Auburn Avenue, Cincinnati, OH 45219, USA
* Corresponding author.
E-mail address: nayak.keshav@scrippshealth.org

Intervent Cardiol Clin 11 (2022) 325–338
https://doi.org/10.1016/j.iccl.2022.03.005
2211-7458/22/© 2022 Published by Elsevier Inc.

- Primary percutaneous coronary intervention (PCI) remains the primary mode of revascularization for patients with STEMI regardless of infection status. A lytic-based strategy is the second-line mode of revascularization at non-PCI capable hospitals or when primary PCI cannot be performed in a timely or safe manner.
- CCL personnel should be vaccinated against SARS-CoV-2. Patients with cardiovascular disease are at an increased risk of severe disease and death from COVID-19 and should be strongly encouraged to be vaccinated, with consideration for booster doses 6 months following their second doses of an mRNA vaccine.
- Like other respiratory viruses (ie, influenza), COVID-19 is strongly associated with an increased risk of acute coronary syndromes and myocardial infarction. All patients presenting for emergency cardiac care should be screened for COVID-19 symptoms and considered for screening by polymerase chain reaction (PCR) testing. Patients presenting for nonurgent, elective procedures should undergo symptom screening before their procedures. During times of high community transmission and in coordination with hospital leadership, PCR testing should be performed within 72 hours of nonurgent, elective procedures; in patients with positive tests, procedures should be delayed at least 10 days when practical and safe. Procedures that cannot be safely delayed should proceed with appropriate infection prevention precautions.

INTRODUCTION

Sterile techniques in the cardiac catheterization laboratory (CCL) have evolved in recent decades, from the days of arterial cutdowns in the 1970s to the current practices of micropuncture percutaneous vessel entry.[1] Percutaneous valve therapy implantation in the hybrid operating room (OR)/CCL has reinforced the importance of strict sterile techniques and infection control protocols. With more than 1 million cardiac catheterization procedures performed annually in the United States,[2] measures in infection control should be standardized to protect both patients and hospital workers.

Recently, the emergent care of patients infected with highly contagious pathogens such as the severe acute respiratory syndrome coronavirus 2 (SARS-CoV-2) has come to the fore. The resulting 2019 coronavirus disease (COVID-19) pandemic initially posed logistical challenges to limiting the spread of aerosolized pathogens until protocols and procedures were implemented to limit infectivity to staff and patients. Ongoing challenges remain as the world faces multiple pandemic waves and novel viral variants. Additionally, the increased risk of acute coronary syndromes and cardiogenic shock require acute management in the CCL due to multiple mechanisms from COVID-19[3] At present, the available evidence-based guidelines do not specifically address CCL preparedness and management of patients in the setting of infectious disease pandemic.[1,4,5] In this review, we seek to specify best practices in the CCL for the management of infected patients in the preprocedure, intraprocedure, and postprocedure environments harmonizing available evidence, recommendations from international heart associations, and consensus opinion.[6–10]

EPIDEMIOLOGY

SARS-CoV-2 is the third highly pathogenic coronavirus to emerge since 2002, following SARS-CoV-2 and the Middle Eastern respiratory syndrome coronavirus (MERS-CoV). Despite genetic and structural similarities to the original SARS virus, SARS-CoV-2 has a lower case-fatality rate but is markedly more contagious, leading to its dramatic spread around the world and high numbers of total deaths, approaching 700,000 in the United States alone and more than 4.7 million deaths worldwide at the time of this writing.[11–13] Total case-fatality rates for COVID-19 are difficult to measure with accuracy given a large number of undiagnosed or minimally symptomatic cases but may be between 1% and 2%. Mortality among hospitalized patients in the US has generally decreased over time but ranges between 8% and 20%, with an increased risk of death noted during major surges when hospital resources are more taxed.[14,15]

The clinical syndromes produced by COVID-19 are well-known at this point. Most of the affected patients experience mild-to-moderate, self-limited respiratory infections.

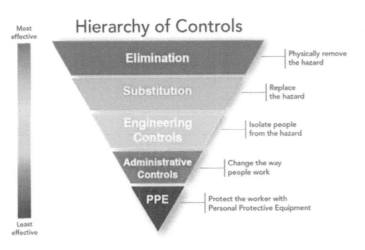

Fig. 1. Levels of infection control in the principles of CCL management.

Patients may be highly contagious and capable of transmitting the virus up to 2 days before symptom onset and for 10 to 21 days afterward, depending on immune status and disease severity.[16] Severe disease, defined as lower respiratory tract infection with oxygen saturation of less than 94% while breathing ambient air, is more common in older adults, those with obesity, or patients with impaired immunity. The most severely affected patients may progress to acute respiratory distress syndrome, shock, and multiorgan failure with an elevated hazard of death.[17] A number of therapies have been evaluated for the treatment of COVID-19, with current guidelines recommending supportive care and monoclonal antibodies for mild-to-moderate disease in high-risk individuals. Antiviral drugs (eg, remdesivir), antithrombotic therapy, glucocorticoids (principally dexamethasone), and immunomodulators such as tocilizumab and baricitinib all play a role in the pharmacologic management of severe disease, depending on illness severity and resource availability.[18]

In late 2020, following an extraordinary global research effort, effective vaccines against SARS-CoV-2 were made available. Multiple vaccine platforms have been studied. The current leading vaccines in the US and worldwide are based on either mRNA platforms, using viral mRNA segments that encode for the SARS-CoV-2 spike protein that are then taken up into the host cytosol, transcribed into their protein products, and then induce a host response and resulting protection; or viral vector platforms, most often a nonreplicating adenovirus that has been modified to encode for the same SARS-CoV-2 spike protein. Three vaccines are currently available in the US (mRNA-1273,

Moderna; BNT162b2, BioNTech-Pfizer; JNJ-78436735, Janssen/Johnson & Johnson). The efficacy of these vaccines against any infection seems to wane over time, in no small part due to the emergence of the highly contagious Delta any Omicron variant, but they remain highly effective at preventing hospitalization and death.[19] In September 2021, the Food and Drug Administration authorized booster doses at 6 months after initial vaccination for high-risk persons, including those 65 years of age or greater, adults with significant medical comorbidities, and those at high risk of occupational exposure (including many health care workers). This was modified in October 2021 to state that boosters may be from any authorized vaccine, not necessarily the specific brand used in the initial vaccination.[20]

PRINCIPLES FOR CARDIAC CATHETERIZATION LABORATORY MANAGEMENT DURING A GLOBAL PANDEMIC

Infection control in the CCL is dependent on careful screening of patients, the availability and proper use of personal protective equipment (PPE), social distancing, administrative and engineering controls (Fig. 1).[10]

HEALTH CARE WORKER PERSONAL PROTECTIVE EQUIPMENT

Protective measures should be taken when treating patients infected with or suspected of infection with pandemic agents. All CCL staff should be provided with PPE, to include N95 respirators, full-face shields, eyewear, disposable fluid impermeable gowns, disposable head caps, surgical gloves, and shoe covers. Proper training for

---

Box 1
Samples steps for donning and doffing personal protective equipment for Cardiac Catheterization Laboratory staff

Donning

1. Tall disposable shoe covers
2. COVID-19 designated lead apron
3. Leaded glasses or prescription glasses
4. First head cover (cover ears)
5. N95 mask
6. Second head cover (cover ears)
7. Surgical mask
8. Eye protection: Goggles or face shield
9. Hand hygiene: Surgical scrub
10. Nonsterile gown
11. Sterile gloves 1
12. Sterile gown
13. Sterile gloves 2

Doffing

1. Hand hygiene (HH1)
2. Remove surgical gown by breaking neck/back straps and dispose sterile gloves
3. HH2 with alcohol foam in room
4. Remove eye protection
5. Remove surgical mask
6. Remove second head cover in room
7. Remove personal protective equipment gown and gloves
8. HH3 with alcohol foam in room
9. Remove shoe covers at doorway in room and step out of room
10. HH4 with alcohol-based disinfectant (ie, Sterillium)
11. Remove N95 mask
12. Remove first head cover
13. HH5 with surgical scrub
14. Remove COVID-19 lead
15. Change to clean scrubs

---

donning and doffing PPE should be carried out with periodic refresher training for CCL staff as outlined in Box 1 and referenced in guidelines, published by the CDC (Fig. 2) as well as by the Infectious Diseases Society of America (IDSA).[9,21,22]

In the setting of a pandemic that may last over several years, stockpiles of PPE should be made available for every wave. When CCL teams perform aerosol-generating procedures (AGP) in patients with suspected or confirmed infections, Powered air-purifying respirators (PAPR) should be worn. Per CDC guidance, AGPs in the CCL include[23]:

1. Open suction of airway secretions
2. Cardiopulmonary resuscitation
3. Endotracheal intubation and extubation
4. Noninvasive positive pressure ventilation (BIPAP, CPAP)
5. Manual ventilation
6. High-flow oxygen delivery

SEQUENCE FOR PUTTING ON
PERSONAL PROTECTIVE EQUIPMENT (PPE)

The type of PPE used will vary based on the level of precautions required, such as standard and contact, droplet or airborne infection isolation precautions. The procedure for putting on and removing PPE should be tailored to the specific type of PPE.

1. GOWN

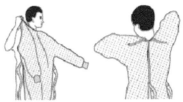

- Fully cover torso from neck to knees, arms to end of wrists, and wrap around the back
- Fasten in back of neck and waist

2. MASK OR RESPIRATOR

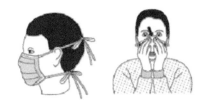

- Secure ties or elastic bands at middle of head and neck
- Fit flexible band to nose bridge
- Fit snug to face and below chin
- Fit-check respirator

3. GOGGLES OR FACE SHIELD

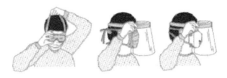

- Place over face and eyes and adjust to fit

4. GLOVES

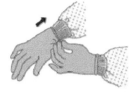

- Extend to cover wrist of isolation gown

USE SAFE WORK PRACTICES TO PROTECT YOURSELF
AND LIMIT THE SPREAD OF CONTAMINATION

- Keep hands away from face
- Limit surfaces touched
- Change gloves when torn or heavily contaminated
- Perform hand hygiene

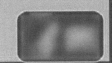

Fig. 2. Sequence for putting on personal protective equipment (PPE).

HEALTH CARE WORKER VACCINATION STATUS

All HCWs should be vaccinated against SARS-CoV-2 to protect themselves, colleagues, and patients. Many health systems in the United States and elsewhere in the world have policies mandating vaccination against COVID-19 for all HCWs. Such mandates have successfully led to vaccine rates in excess of 90% in affected staff.

HOW TO SAFELY REMOVE PERSONAL PROTECTIVE EQUIPMENT (PPE) EXAMPLE 1

There are a variety of ways to safely remove PPE without contaminating your clothing, skin, or mucous membranes with potentially infectious materials. Here is one example. **Remove all PPE before exiting the patient room except a respirator, if worn. Remove the respirator after leaving the patient room and closing the door.** Remove PPE in the following sequence:

1. GLOVES

- Outside of gloves are contaminated!
- If your hands get contaminated during glove removal, immediately wash your hands or use an alcohol-based hand sanitizer
- Using a gloved hand, grasp the palm area of the other gloved hand and peel off first glove
- Hold removed glove in gloved hand
- Slide fingers of ungloved hand under remaining glove at wrist and peel off second glove over first glove
- Discard gloves in a waste container

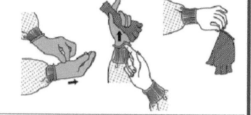

2. GOGGLES OR FACE SHIELD

- Outside of goggles or face shield are contaminated!
- If your hands get contaminated during goggle or face shield removal, immediately wash your hands or use an alcohol-based hand sanitizer
- Remove goggles or face shield from the back by lifting head band or ear pieces
- If the item is reusable, place in designated receptacle for reprocessing. Otherwise, discard in a waste container

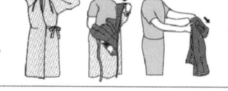

3. GOWN

- Gown front and sleeves are contaminated!
- If your hands get contaminated during gown removal, immediately wash your hands or use an alcohol-based hand sanitizer
- Unfasten gown ties, taking care that sleeves don't contact your body when reaching for ties
- Pull gown away from neck and shoulders, touching inside of gown only
- Turn gown inside out
- Fold or roll into a bundle and discard in a waste container

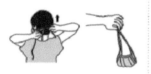

4. MASK OR RESPIRATOR

- Front of mask/respirator is contaminated — DO NOT TOUCH!
- If your hands get contaminated during mask/respirator removal, immediately wash your hands or use an alcohol-based hand sanitizer
- Grasp bottom ties or elastics of the mask/respirator, then the ones at the top, and remove without touching the front
- Discard in a waste container

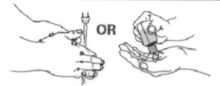

5. WASH HANDS OR USE AN ALCOHOL-BASED HAND SANITIZER IMMEDIATELY AFTER REMOVING ALL PPE

OR

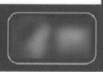

PERFORM HAND HYGIENE BETWEEN STEPS IF HANDS BECOME CONTAMINATED AND IMMEDIATELY AFTER REMOVING ALL PPE

Fig. 2. *(continued)*

Despite early concerns regarding mass resignations, rates of staff dismissed due to vaccine noncompliance have been low, often less than 1% of HCWs.[24] Reasons for medical exemptions are rare and should be reviewed with the best available medical evidence, the risks of immunization weighed against the risk of morbidity and mortality to the staff member from

HOW TO SAFELY REMOVE PERSONAL PROTECTIVE EQUIPMENT (PPE) EXAMPLE 2

Here is another way to safely remove PPE without contaminating your clothing, skin, or mucous membranes with potentially infectious materials. Remove all PPE before exiting the patient room except a respirator, if worn. Remove the respirator after leaving the patient room and closing the door. Remove PPE in the following sequence:

1. GOWN AND GLOVES

- Gown front and sleeves and the outside of gloves are contaminated!
- If your hands get contaminated during gown or glove removal, immediately wash your hands or use an alcohol-based hand sanitizer
- Grasp the gown in the front and pull away from your body so that the ties break, touching outside of gown only with gloved hands
- While removing the gown, fold or roll the gown inside-out into a bundle
- As you are removing the gown, peel off your gloves at the same time, only touching the inside of the gloves and gown with your bare hands. Place the gown and gloves into a waste container

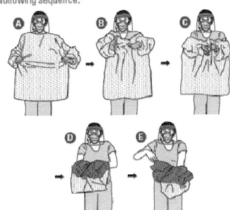

2. GOGGLES OR FACE SHIELD

- Outside of goggles or face shield are contaminated!
- If your hands get contaminated during goggle or face shield removal, immediately wash your hands or use an alcohol-based hand sanitizer
- Remove goggles or face shield from the back by lifting head band and without touching the front of the goggles or face shield
- If the item is reusable, place in designated receptacle for reprocessing. Otherwise, discard in a waste container

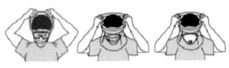

3. MASK OR RESPIRATOR

- Front of mask/respirator is contaminated — DO NOT TOUCH!
- If your hands get contaminated during mask/respirator removal, immediately wash your hands or use an alcohol-based hand sanitizer
- Grasp bottom ties or elastics of the mask/respirator, then the ones at the top, and remove without touching the front
- Discard in a waste container

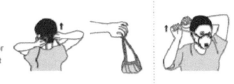

4. WASH HANDS OR USE AN ALCOHOL-BASED HAND SANITIZER IMMEDIATELY AFTER REMOVING ALL PPE

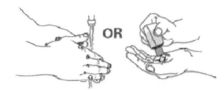

OR

PERFORM HAND HYGIENE BETWEEN STEPS IF HANDS BECOME CONTAMINATED AND IMMEDIATELY AFTER REMOVING ALL PPE

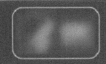

Fig. 2. (continued)

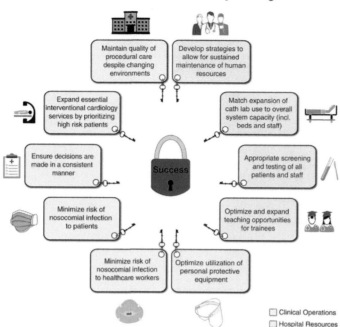

Successful Cath Lab Reboot Key Strategies

- Maintain quality of procedural care despite changing environments
- Develop strategies to allow for sustained maintenance of human resources
- Expand essential interventional cardiology services by prioritizing high risk patients
- Match expansion of cath lab use to overall system capacity (incl. beds and staff)
- Ensure decisions are made in a consistent manner
- Appropriate screening and testing of all patients and staff
- Minimize risk of nosocomial infection to patients
- Optimize and expand teaching opportunities for trainees
- Minimize risk of nosocomial infection to healthcare workers
- Optimize utilization of personal protective equipment

Success

☐ Clinical Operations
☐ Hospital Resources

Fig. 3. Guiding principles for successful catheterization laboratory reboot.[30]

COVID-19, and the need to protect vulnerable patients from infection.

ENVIRONMENTAL/ENGINEERING CONTROLS

Hospital facilities departments and leadership should devise an overarching plan to limit aerosol transmission in procedural areas. Facilities should test the positive pressure ventilation systems of the CCL and verify OR conditions to ensure proper functioning air-handling units with adequate air exchange rate, room differential pressure, relative humidity, and air temperature. If possible, hospitals should isolate a single CCL or operating room for patients presumed or confirmed to be infected with COVID-19. Furthermore, modification of ventilation systems should be considered to eliminate the virus from the operating room environment in an expeditious manner. If available, negative pressure ventilation rooms can be designated as the "COVID-19 operating room," thereby providing the ideal protection to health care personnel in adjoining operating rooms or corridors. In some instances, departments have been able to convert existing CCLs into negative pressure rooms temporarily.[25] Most importantly, doors of the CCL should remain closed at all times during the procedure. Opening

doors could result in loss of positive room pressure and cause viral burden in the air to be dispersed out of the CCL and cross-contaminate adjoining areas, corridors, or even the adjacent operating room.[26,27]

To preserve optimal clean airflow into the CCL or operating room, an OR should have an air exchange rate of greater than or equal to 20 times the room volume in an hour.[28] An air exchange rate lower than that will increase the viral burden in the environment due to stagnant airflow. There are standard calculations for air exchange depending on the pressurization of the operating room. In a positive pressure OR, the following calculation can be made[29]:

Air exchange per hour = Total supply air (m³/min) x 60 divided by Room volume (m³)

Once adequate air exchanges are confirmed, positive pressurization of the rooms should be confirmed compared with adjoining areas thereby creating the proper barrier between the OR doors to prevent dispersion of airborne viral particles.

ADMINISTRATIVE CONTROLS

Only CCL personnel and health care workers involved in the procedure for presumed or confirmed patients with COVID-19 should be permitted inside the CCL. As always, the CCL

Table 1
Classification of interventional procedures according to their indication during the Coronavirus disease 2019 pandemic

Category[a]	Coronary Angiography/PCI	Structural Intervention	Peripheral Anglography/PVI

I	• Class III/IV angina despite medical therapy
	• Recent hospitalization for angina/NSTEMI
	• High-risk stress
	  o Drop in BP with exercise (>10 mm Hg)
	  o Angina at low effort
	  o Sustained VT
	  o ST-segment elevation
	  o Drop in LVEF
	  o TID on imaging
	  o Large Ischemic burden
		• TAVR: severe AS or bioprosthetic failure with
		  o Class IV symptoms
		  o Recurrent or refractory heart failure requiring hospitalization
		  o Decline in LVEF
		  o Syncope
		• Percutaneous mitral valve repair/replacement
		  o Refractory to medical therapy while inpatient
		• Acute post-MI VSD
			• Critical limb ischemia with rest pain/nonhealing ulcer
			• Endovascular repair of symptomatic AAA or enlarging TAA
			• Nonfunctioning dialysis fistula
			• Acute iliofemoral DVT with concern for phlegmasia
			• Acute pulmonary embolism with corpulmonale

II	• Class II angina despite maximal medical therapy
	• Abnormal stress test result without high-risk feature
	• Pre-TAVR or cardiothoracic procedure
	• Pretransplantation evaluation (cardiac or other)
	• Pulmonary hypertension evaluation
		• Progressive or escalating symptoms (Class III/IV) or recent hospitalization for heart failure (<30 d>)
		  o TAVR
		  o Percutaneous mitral valve repair/replacement
		  o Percutaneous pulmonary valve repair/replacement
		  o Percutaneous tricuspid valve repair/replacement
		• Severe AS with mean gradient >60 mm Hg or peak velocity >5 m/s
		• Severe MR with recent decline in LVEF
			• Progressive or escalating claudication (limb or abdominal)
			• Endovascular repair of enlarging AAA or IAA
			• Symptomatic carotid stenosis
			• IVC filter placement for acute DVT

III	• CTO case
	• CardioMEMS implantation
		• Stable symptoms (Class II) or asymptomatic with an indication for intervention
		  o TAVR
		  o Mitral valve repair/replacement
		  o Pulmonary valve replacement
		• ASD/PFO closure
		• LAA occlusion
		• PDA closure
		• Chronic VSD closure
		• Alcohol septal ablation
			• All stable symptomatic PAD
			• Chronic venous disease
			• IVC filter removal

Abbreviations: AAA, abdominal aortic aneurysm; AS, aortic stenosis; ASD, atrial septal defect; BP, blood pressure; CTO, chronic total occlusion; DVT, deep vein thrombosis; IVC, inferior vena cava; LAA, left ductus appendage; LVEF, left ventricular ejection fraction; MI, myocardial infarction; NSTEMI, non-ST segment elevation infarction; PCI, percutaneous coronary intervention; PDA, patent ductus arteriosus; PFO, patent foramen ovale; PVI, peripheral vascular intervention; TAA, thoracic aortic aneurysm; TABR, transcatheter aortic valve replacement; TID, transient ischemic dilatation; VSD, ventricular septal defect; VT, ventricular tachycardia.

[a] Category I (urgent procedure): patient at high risk for CV complications while waiting; Category II (semiurgent procedure): at moderate CV risk; category III (elective): at low CV risk.

door should remain closed at all times during the procedure. All necessary equipment should be stored within the CCL to avoid the opening of the CCL doors to procure supplies. All nonessential personnel such as vendors or visitors should be prohibited from entering the CCL during procedures for presumed or confirmed patients with COVID-19.

Table 2
Phased-in model for restarting interventional elective procedures during the COVID-19 pandemic

Phases	Cases	Dependencies	Tactics
Phase 1: urgent/ emergent procedures and those not affecting surge resources 25% usual capacity	1. Category I patients 2. Patients who have been waiting >4 wk	1. Nursing staff to open procedure room to accept elective outpatients 2. "Clean" waiting area 3. "Clean" area of overnight stay 4. Equipment removed to support other areas 5. Recover TAVR and high-risk patients in the procedure room 6. Availability of cardiac anesthesia and cardiac surgery 7. ICU bed availability	1. Return of 25% of catheterization laboratory nurse FTEs 2. Physicians review patient list to identify priority patients 3. No visitors 4. Greeter to escort through a separate entrance 5. Direct to room/social distancing 6. Open holding area or dedicated overnight stay area. 7. Anesthesia machines, procedure tables, and equipment carts reclaimed 8. Testing all outpatients prior to arrival 9. COVID-19 procedure room for patients 10. Careful patient selection to reduce the likelihood of needing ICU bed 11. Cluster procedure types
Phase II: semiurgent procedures, possibility affecting surge resources 50% usual capacity	1. Category I and II patients 2. Patients who have been waiting >3 wk	As above 1. Holding area space reopened for pre/ postprocedural care 2. Staffing and room availability 3. Throughput	As above 1. Universal COVID-19 testing for patients 2. Continue to isolate high-risk population to reduce exposure 3. Adequate staffing for cases (nursing and technologist) 4. Adequate staffing to provide pre/ postprocedural care 5. Return of 1 FTE for environmental services and patient transport
Phase III: routine procedures 75% usual capacity	1. Category I, II, and III patients 2. Patients who have been waiting >2 wk	As above 1. Staffing and room availability 2. Throughput	As above 1. Return of 80% FTEs to procedural area including transport, environmental services, and catheterization laboratory and holding area nursing

(continued on next page)

Phases	Cases	Dependencies	Tactics
Table 2 *(continued)*			
Phase 4: 110% of FY20 budgeted procedural cases	1. Category I, II, and III patients	As above 1. Staffing and room availability 2. Throughput	As above 1. Running 1 procedure room on saturday 2. Reestabilish all blocks for ORs and anesthesia support 3. Return of all clinical/ nonclinical staff members to procedural and pre/ postprocedural care areas 4. Seek additional blocks as needed

Abbreviations: COVID-19, Coronavirus disease 2019, FTE, full-time equivalent; FY20, fiscal year 2020; ICU, intensive care unit; OR, operating room; TAVR, transcatheter aortic valve replacement.

REOPENING CARDIAC CATHETERIZATION LABORATORY SAFELY FOR ELECTIVE CASE SCHEDULING

With gradual recovery from the peak of the COVID-19 pandemic, CCL have safely resumed elective cardiovascular procedures with continued guiding Principles to limit the risk of exposure of CCL health care workers to patients with active COVID-19 infection. Central to these principles is the testing of all patients with a single swab 24 to 48 hours before their elective procedure. In the event this preliminary test is positive, the patient is instructed to self-isolate and reschedule their elective procedure in 10 to 14 days with the confirmation of a negative test. Successful strategies for CCL recovery are outlined in **Fig. 3**, **Tables 1–3**[30] with proper case selection.[31,32]

SUMMARY

The severe acute respiratory syndrome coronavirus-2 (SARS-CoV-2) is a highly contagious pathogen leading to its dramatic spread around the world and high numbers of total deaths, approaching 700,000 in the United States and more than 4.7 million deaths worldwide. CCL teams are frontline workers and should be provided with N95 respirators, whole face shields or protective eyewear, disposable caps, shoe covers, sterile gowns, and surgical gloves. The CCL needs formal preparedness protocols in the form of consensus evidence-based guidance and guidelines from international heart associations. All CCL personnel should be vaccinated against SARS-CoV-2 along with timely booster vaccinations. Patients with cardiovascular disease are at an increased risk of severe disease and death from COVID-19 and should be strongly encouraged to be vaccinated, with consideration for booster doses 6 months following their second doses of an mRNA vaccine. Like other respiratory viruses (ie, influenza), COVID-19 is strongly associated with an increased risk of acute coronary syndromes and myocardial infarction. All patients presenting for emergency cardiac care should be screened for COVID-19 symptoms and considered for screening by polymerase chain reaction (PCR) testing. During times of high community transmission and in coordination with hospital leadership, PCR testing should be performed within 72 hours of nonurgent, elective procedures; in patients with positive tests, procedures should be delayed at least 10 days when practical and safe. Procedures that cannot be safely delayed should proceed with appropriate infection prevention precautions.

Further research characterizing the effectiveness of implemented measures during the COVID-19 pandemic so that caregivers and medical institutions can understand the logistics of implementing policies. Iterative improvements to minimize the transmission of pathogens, particularly aerosolized microorganisms, should be disseminated and routinely reviewed as part of the contingency policies of CCL for future pandemics.

Table 3
Specific considerations for structural heart procedures during the COVID-19 pandemic

Procedure	Procedural Considerations	Operational Considerations
TAVR	• MAC or conscious sedation (avoid general anesthesia) • Early permanent pacemaker implantation for advanced heart blocks seen Post-TAVR • Same-day discharge in low-risk patients with home cardiac monitoring	• Dedicated COVID-19-negative pathway (pre and postprocedure) • Only essential team present in the room (8) • Same-day or next-day discharge • Discharge home (not to a rehabilitation center or nursing home) • Crash ICU bed available • Telehealth for pre and postprocedural visits
MitraClip	• No preprocedural TEE (diagnostic imaging obtained during the case)	
ASD/PFO closure	• No preprocedural TEE (imaging obtained during the case) • ICE for procedural guidance (avoid TEE)	
LAAO	• No preprocedural TEE • ICE for procedural guidance (avoid TEE)	

Abbreviations: ICE, intracardiac echocardiography; LAAO, left atrial appendage occlusion; MAC, monitored anesthesia; PTEE, transesophageal echocardiography; other abbreviations as in Tables 1 and 2.

CLINICS CARE POINTS

- All CCL staff should be provided with PPE, to include N95 respirators, full-face shields, eyewear, disposable fluid impermeable gowns, disposable head caps, surgical gloves, and shoe covers
- Proper training for donning and doffing PPE should be carried out with periodic refresher training for CCL staff
- Primary percutaneous coronary intervention (PCI) remains the primary mode of revascularization for patients with STEMI regardless of infection status
- All HCWs should be vaccinated against SARS-CoV-2 to protect themselves, colleagues, and patients
- Only CCL personnel and health care workers involved in the procedure for presumed or confirmed patients with COVID-19 should be permitted inside the CCL
- To limit the risk of exposure of CCL health care workers to patients with active COVID-19 infection, testing of all patients with a single swab 24 to 48 hours before their elective procedure is recommended.

DISCLOSURE

The authors have nothing to disclose.

REFERENCES

1. Chambers CE, Eisenhauer MD, McNicol LB, et al. Members of the Catheterization Lab Performance Standards Committee for the Society for Cardiovascular Angiography and Interventions. Infection control guidelines for the cardiac catheterization laboratory: society guidelines revisited. Catheter Cardiovasc Interv 2006;67(1):78–86.

2. Virani SS, Alonso A, Benjamin EJ, et al. American Heart Association Council on Epidemiology and Prevention Statistics Committee and Stroke Statistics Subcommittee. Heart Disease and Stroke Statistics-2020 Update: A Report From the American Heart Association. Circulation 2020;141(9): e139–596.

3. Chew NWS, Ow ZGW, Teo VXY, et al. The Global Effect of the COVID-19 Pandemic on STEMI Care: A Systematic Review and Meta-analysis. Can J Cardiol 2021;37(9):1450–9.

4. Bangalore S, Barsness GW, Dangas GD, et al. Evidence-Based Practices in the Cardiac Catheterization Laboratory: A Scientific Statement From the American Heart Association. Circulation 2021; 144(5):e107–19.

5. Naidu SS, Abbott JD, Bagai J, et al. SCAI expert consensus update on best practices in the cardiac catheterization laboratory: This statement was endorsed by the American College of Cardiology (ACC), the American Heart Association (AHA), and the Heart Rhythm Society (HRS) in April 2021. Catheter Cardiovasc Interv 2021;98(2):255–76.

6. FGP Welt, Shah PB, Aronow HD, et al. American College of Cardiology's Interventional Council and the Society for Cardiovascular Angiography and Interventions. Catheterization Laboratory Considerations During the Coronavirus (COVID-19) Pandemic: From the ACC's Interventional Council and SCAI. J Am Coll Cardiol 2020;75(18):2372–5.

7. Mahmud E, Dauerman HL, FGP Welt, et al. Management of Acute Myocardial Infarction During the COVID-19 Pandemic: A Position Statement From the Society for Cardiovascular Angiography and Interventions (SCAI), the American College of Cardiology (ACC), and the American College of Emergency Physicians (ACEP). J Am Coll Cardiol 2020;76(11):1375–84.

8. European Society for Cardiology. ESC guidance for the diagnosis and management of CV disease during the COVID-19 pandemic. 2020. Available at: https://www.escardio.org/Education/COVID-19-and-Cardioloft/ESC-COVID-19-Guidance. Accessed November 1, 2020.

9. Szerlip M, Anwaruddin S, Aronow HD, et al. Considerations for cardiac catheterization laboratory procedures during the COVID-19 pandemic perspectives from the Society for Cardiovascular Angiography and Interventions Emerging Leader Mentorship (SCAI ELM) Members and Graduates. Catheter Cardiovasc Interv 2020;96(3):586–97.

10. Tsui KL, Li SK, Li MC, et al. Preparedness of the cardiac catheterization laboratory for severe acute respiratory syndrome (SARS) and other epidemics. J Invasive Cardiol 2005;17(3):149–52.

11. Rossi GA, Sacco O, Mancino E, et al. Differences and similarities between SARS-CoV and SARS-CoV-2: spike receptor-binding domain recognition and host cell infection with support of cellular serine proteases. Infection 2020;48(5):665–9.

12. Available at: https://covid.cdc.gov/covid-data-tracker/#datatracker-home. Accessed October 03, 2021.

13. Available at: https://covid19.who.int/. Accessed October 03, 2021.

14. Finelli L, Gupta V, Petigara T, et al. Mortality Among US Patients Hospitalized With SARS-CoV-2 Infection in 2020. JAMA Netw Open 2021;4(4): e216556.

15. Kadri SS, Sun J, Lawandi A, et al. Association Between Caseload Surge and COVID-19 Survival in 558 U.S. Hospitals, March to August 2020. Ann Intern Med 2021;174(9):1240–51.

16. Lynch JB, Davitkov P, Anderson DJ, et al. Infectious Diseases Society of America Guidelines on Infection Prevention for Health Care Personnel Caring for Patients with Suspected or Known COVID-19. Clin Infect Dis 2020. https://doi.org/10.1093/cid/ciaa1063. ciaa1063.

17. Berlin DA, Gulick RM, Martinez FJ. Severe Covid-19. N Engl J Med 2020;383(25):2451–60.

18. Available at. https://www.covid19treatmentguide-lines.nih.gov/. Accessed October 03, 2021.

19. Self WH, Tenforde MW, Rhoads JP, et al, IVY Network. Comparative Effectiveness of Moderna, Pfizer-BioNTech, and Janssen (Johnson & Johnson) Vaccines in Preventing COVID-19 Hospitalizations Among Adults Without Immunocompromising Conditions - United States, March-August 2021. MMWR Morb Mortal Wkly Rep 2021;70(38):1337–43.

20. Available at: https://www.fda.gov/news-events/press-announcements/coronavirus-covid-19-update-fda-takes-additional-actions-use-booster-dose-covid-19-vaccines. Accessed November 1, 2021.

21. Lynch JB, Davitkov P, Anderson DJ, et al. Infectious Diseases Society of America Guidelines on Infection Prevention for Healthcare Personnel Caring for Patients with Suspected or Known COVID-19. Clin Infect Dis 2021. https://doi.org/10.1093/cid/ciab953. ciab953.

22. Johm T-J, Hassan K, Weich H. Donning and doffing of personal protective equipment (PPE) for angiography during the COVID-19 Crisis. Eur Heart J 2020. https://doi.org/10.1093/eurheartj/ehaa283. ehaa283.

23. CDC reference health.state.mn.us 6/22/21.

24. Dyer O. Covid-19: New York's health workers agree to vaccinate as mandate bites. BMJ 2021;374: n2390.

25. Chow TT, Kwan A, Lin Z, et al. Conversion of operating theatre from positive to negative pressure environment. J Hosp Infect 2006;64(4):371–8.

26. Mckenna K, Hutchinson A, Butler M. An evaluation of the environmental factors that impact on operating room air quality and the risk for development of surgical site infections. Infect Dis Health 2019;24:S7.

27. Sadrizadeh S, Pantelic J, Sherman M, et al. Airborne particle dispersion to an operating room environment during sliding and hinged door opening. Abouali O J Infect Public Health 2018;11(5): 631–5.

28. Standard ISO. ISO 14644-1, Cleanrooms and associated controlled environments, Classification of air cleanliness. United Kingdom: Institute of Environmental Sciences and Technology; 1999.

29. Standard NEBB. Procedural standards for certified testing of cleanrooms, adjusting and balancing of environmental systems. USA: National Environmental Balancing Bureau; 2009.

30. Poulin MF, Pinto DS. Strategies for Successful Catheterization Laboratory Recovery From the COVID-19 Pandemic. JACC Cardiovasc Interv 2020;13(16):1951–7.

31. Vemmou E, Nikolakopoulos I, Brilakis ES, et al. Case Selection During the COVID-19 Pandemic: Who Should Go to the Cardiac Catheterization Laboratory? Curr Treat Options Cardiovasc Med 2021;23(4):27.

32. Zaman M, Tiong D, Saw J, et al. Sustainable Resumption of Cardiac Catheterization Laboratory Procedures, and the Importance of Testing, During Endemic COVID-19. Curr Treat Options Cardiovasc Med 2021;23(3):22.

Acute Neurointervention for Ischemic Stroke

Owais Khadem Alsrouji, MBBS[a], Alex Bou Chebl, MD, FSVIN[b],*

KEYWORDS

• Stroke • LVO • Mechanical thrombectomy

KEY POINTS

- Advent and implementation of stent retrievers has revolutionized the management of ischemic strokes caused by large vessel occlusion (LVO).
- Patient selection is complex. Salient variables for case selection include patient age, prestroke disability, National Institutes of Health Stroke Scale score, LVO territory/location, and time of presentation from symptom onset.
- Quality of reperfusion after the first pass of mechanical thrombectomy is associated with better outcomes.

INTRODUCTION

Acute ischemic stroke (AIS) remains one of the major causes of death worldwide and a leading cause of disability. Historically, stroke care has been very challenging, and only recently has major progress been made in improving neurologic outcomes and reducing mortality. A major obstacle to advances in stroke care has been the delayed recognition of stroke symptoms by the lay public as well as clinicians. In addition, the risk of intracranial hemorrhage (ICH) due to revascularization therapies has been the major hurdle to improving stroke outcomes. It is the most feared complication of AIS therapy and when it occurs in this setting it is often catastrophic and essentially untreatable. This risk was very high with early trials of a variety of thrombolytic agents. It was not until 1995 that the first proven treatment of AIS, intravenous tissue plasminogen activator, was confirmed. That treatment was of marginal benefit, and it would take another 20 years before a highly effective treatment of the most severe strokes, large vessel occlusions (LVO), would be validated. This endovascular therapy (EVT), also known as mechanical embolectomy, requires the prompt recognition of stroke symptoms, rapid imaging of the cerebrum and the cerebral vasculature often with advanced imaging of the ischemic penumbra. Once the appropriate patient is selected to minimize the risk of ICH and maximize the potential benefit, then treatment must be initiated quickly to reduce stroke morbidity and mortality.

LARGE VESSEL OCCLUSION, DEFINITION, AND PATHOPHYSIOLOGY

AIS due to LVO is defined as the abrupt neurologic dysfunction caused by a disruption of the arterial blood supply by an occlusion of a cervical or intracranial artery. This occlusion can be in the anterior circulation (ie, internal carotid territory) or posterior circulation (ie, vertebra-basilar territory). LVO accounts for about 30% of all AIS.[1] Cause of LVO can be cardioembolic, thromboembolic (ie, artery to artery), atherosclerotic with in-situ thrombosis, and lastly cryptogenic when no clear cause is identified. The management approach is generally the same in the acute phase regardless of the cause.

[a] Department of Neurosurgery, Henry Ford Hospital, K11, 2799 West Grand Boulevard, Detroit, MI 48202, USA;
[b] Division of Vascular Neurology, Department of Neurology, Harris Comprehensive Stroke Center, Henry Ford Health System, Clara Ford Pavillion, Room 453, 2799 W Grand Boulevard, Detroit, MI 48202, USA
* Corresponding author.
E-mail address: achebl1@hfhs.org

Intervent Cardiol Clin 11 (2022) 339–347
https://doi.org/10.1016/j.iccl.2022.03.006
2211-7458/22/© 2022 Elsevier Inc. All rights reserved.

CLINICAL PRESENTATION AND EARLY DETECTION

In LVO stroke, every 1 minute of ischemia destroys about 1.9 million neurons and 14 billion synapses[2]; this makes early recognition and prompt revascularization crucial. Recognition of LVO strokes starts in the prehospital setting with emergency medical services. Various scores have been developed to help recognize LVO stroke and categorize its severity. These scores can facilitate communication with stroke centers before arrival. Although many scores have been developed, none have been shown to be superior to others and they all share a focus on the presence of motor and cortical symptoms. Regardless of the score used, LVO stroke should be suspected when a patient shows cortical signs (Box 1). The presence of cortical signs is a good indicator for anterior circulation LVO stroke in the prehospital as well as in-hospital setting.[3] The detection of posterior circulation strokes remains challenging due to their relative rarity (approximately 10% of LVO) but also due to the myriad clinical symptoms as well as the higher likelihood of slow clinical progression and alteration of consciousness, which can often be misdiagnosed as "confusion" or "encephalopathy."

PATIENT SELECTION AND IMAGING IN THE ACUTE PHASE

All patients presenting with strokelike symptoms should undergo a computed tomography (CT) scan of the head without contrast to exclude ICH. The presence of ICH is generally a contraindication to revascularization therapy for AIS. Often LVO can be suspected on clinical grounds if there are signs of cortical ischemia or a high National Institutes of Health Stroke Scale (NIHSS)—the latter is the standard research and clinical scale for defining stroke severity. The scale gives patients points for deficits, and the score can range from 0 for patients who are nearly normal to 42 for those who are comatose and moribund. A score of 7 or more has been found to have a positive predictive value for LVO of 84.2%.[4] The higher the score, the more severe the stroke and the greater the thrombus burden. On imaging with CT head without contrast, a hyperdense vessel sign can be seen, and this can also suggest the presence of an LVO (Fig. 1). However, the gold standard for acute phase confirmation of LVO is CT angiography (CTA) of the head and neck, which is used to select the most appropriate candidates for EVT. A recent single-center study revealed increase in LVO detection with performing CTA for all patients presenting with strokelike symptoms with decrease in the door to groin time and a signal toward favorable clinical outcomes.[5] Furthermore, head and neck vessel imaging have been the standard of care for stroke etiology workup. Hence, our practice has been to perform CTA head and neck in addition to CT head in the acute phase for all patients presenting with strokelike symptoms. An alternative approach in case of limited resources is to perform CTA only for patients with high suspicion for LVO such as those with a high NIHSS. The American Heart/Stroke Association (AHA/ASA) guidelines for endovascular treatment of LVO recommends that the NIHSS be 6 or higher. Patients with LVO in the posterior circulation may not show cortical signs/symptoms but rather cranial nerve deficits, motor symptoms, and/or decreased level of alertness.

In addition to the aforementioned criteria, many other clinical criteria must be considered in deciding who is a candidate for revascularization therapy. Baseline blood pressure, glucose levels, the use of anticoagulants, recent stroke symptoms or neurosurgical procedures, baseline cognitive function and level of independence, age, and many others may all affect the risk of ICH with revascularization as well as the potential for clinical benefit. More controversial is the use of advanced imaging techniques such as perfusion imaging to determine eligibility. CT perfusion (CTP) imaging is the most commonly used and is able to determine the presence of a completed infarct (infarct core) as well as regions of critical hypoperfusion, which are still salvageable (ischemic penumbra). Proponents feel that CTP imaging increases the probability of identifying patients who would benefit from treatment, as revascularization of a completed infarct is of no benefit to the patient and only increases the risk of harm. Opponents of CTP argue that the time delay in obtaining and interpreting the studies is unnecessary and only serves the purpose of excluding patients from treatment. They feel a clinical-CT mismatch (ie, a severe clinical deficit with no to minimal signs of early infarct on CT) is comparable to CTP imaging. This issue is currently unresolved but it is hoped that ongoing clinical trials would bring clarity soon.

More recently multiple artificial intelligence software platforms have been developed for the automatic detection of LVO and CTP deficits. Several have received Food and Drug Administration (FDA) approval for clinical use.

These platforms can be installed on the CT scanner and within minutes of image acquisition can send out email and smart phone notifications of the presence of an LVO. Although not perfect, their sensitivity and specificity are high enough (>80% for both) that they are increasingly becoming the standard means of LVO and ischemic penumbra detection especially when specialized neuroradiological interpretation is not emergently available.

THROMBOLYSIS THERAPY

Recombinant Tissue Plasminogen Activator

Intravenous recombinant tissue plasminogen activator (rtPA) remains the standard of care for patients presenting with AIS within 3 to 4.5 hours of symptom onset including patients with LVO. The use of intravenous (IV) tPA is limited to patients who meet specific and extensive criteria aimed at minimizing the risk of ICH. It is dosed 0.9 mg/kg with a maximum dosage of 90 mg; 10% is given as a bolus, and the remainder is infused over 1 hour. rtPA is most effective in patients presenting within 60 minutes of symptom onset and in those with a smaller thrombus burden. The site and size of the thrombus influences recanalization rates after rtPA with more proximal occlusions, for example, internal carotid artery, the least likely to recanalize.[6–8] As with facilitated thrombolysis in patients with ST segment elevation myocardial infarction there has been debate as to whether IV thrombolysis is of utility in the modern era of EVT. Two trials from China and Japan (DIRECT-MT, SKIP) demonstrated noninferiority of EVT with mechanical thrombectomy (MT) alone compared with MT plus intravenous rtPA for functional outcome. However, DIRECT-MT did show that MT alone was associated with significantly lower recanalization. Conversely, combination treatment showed higher rates of symptomatic ICH.[9,10] A meta-analysis of 30 studies showed better clinical outcomes, lower mortality at 90 days, and higher successful recanalization rates, without increasing the risk of hemorrhagic complications with combination therapy.[11] Because EVT is not always feasible or can fail to reach the site of occlusion, in keeping with AHA/ASA guidelines, our practice has been to administer rtPA to all those who qualify in combination with MT, especially if the patient is being transferred from a primary stroke center to a thrombectomy capable center.[12]

Tenecteplase

The use of tenecteplase in AIS remains a hot topic for discussion, given that IV rtPA is the only FDA-approved treatment of AIS to date. Tenecteplase, a genetically engineered mutant form of rtPA has been studied as a possible alternative to rtPA because of its longer half-life and higher fibrin specificity; the latter may be associated with lower risks of bleeding. It is also more convenient to administer as an intravenous single bolus as compared with rtPA that requires a bolus followed by an hour-long infusion. A meta-analysis of the major trials (ATTEST and EXTEND-IA TNK) in patients with LVOs showed higher odds of successful recanalization and good functional outcomes with tenecteplase compared with rtPA.[13] Although the optimal dose of tenecteplase for AIS remains unknown, current AHA/ASA guidelines consider tenecteplase (0.25 mg/kg dose with a maximum dose of 25mg) a reasonable alternative for patients undergoing thrombectomy.[12] TNK-S2B trial is currently enrolling to identify the optimal dose of tenecteplase with comparison to rtPA.

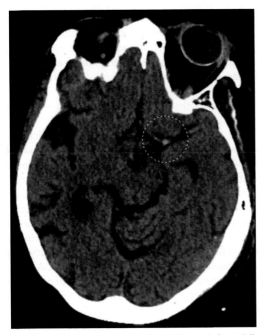

Fig. 1. Circle pointing out a hyperdense left middle cerebral artery suggesting an occlusion.

MECHANICAL THROMBECTOMY

Initial approaches to the endovascular treatment of AIS consisted of intraarterial thrombolysis with marginal clinical benefits and high complication rates.[14,15] The first FDA-approved device for AIS treatment was the MERCI (Concentric Medical Inc., CA, USA) retriever device of the early 2000s followed by the and Penumbra Inc. aspiration system. Although both devices had variable success in cerebral thrombectomy, these systems failed to show superiority over IV rtPA alone in 3 different trials published in 2013 (IMS-III, MR RESCUE, SYNTHESIS).[14–16] A breakthrough in the management for LVO stroke was the advent of the so-called stent retrievers. These devices consist of self-expanding (nitinol) stents permanently attached to 0.014″ wires. They are deployed within the occlusion/thrombus and removed a few minutes later after the thrombus has been integrated within their interstices. They are often used with a balloon occlusion guide catheter, which is used to occlude antegrade flow and permit the creation of a suction effect while the device is removed, facilitating thrombus removal.

MT has been studied primarily in patients with anterior circulation LVO. The anterior circulation includes the internal carotid (ICA), middle cerebral (MCA), and anterior cerebral arteries (ACA). The posterior circulation includes the vertebral, basilar (BA), and posterior cerebral arteries.

PATIENT SELECTION FOR MECHANICAL THROMBECTOMY IN ANTERIOR CIRCULATION LARGE VESSEL OCCLUSION

Based on the available clinical trials, careful selection of patients for mechanical thrombectomy is crucial for good outcomes. The following aspects must be taken into consideration when selecting patients:

Age Less Than or Equal to 18 Years

The available randomized controlled trials included patients who were 18 years and older. However, good neurologic outcome has been reported in case series and meta-analysis of pediatric age group who received mechanical thrombectomy.[17] In its recent report the Society of Neurointerventional Surgery recommends against withholding mechanical thrombectomy from the pediatric age group.[18] On the other end of the spectrum, the very old (90 years and older) do not have as good of outcomes as younger patients; however, all studies have shown a consistently high relative benefit for

this population mostly because lack of recanalization is associated with almost uniformly poor outcomes.

Prestroke Disability

Good baseline functional status prestroke was one of the inclusion criteria for most of the clinical trials in the early and extended time windows; this was defined as a Modified Rankin Scale (mRS) score of 0 or 1 (Table 1), that is, patients with moderate or severe disabilities were excluded. Data from good, randomized trials are lacking for this patient population. Retrospective studies have shown mixed results in terms of good outcomes or return to baseline.[19,20] AHA/ASA guidelines support treatment of patients with independent baseline function, that is, mRS 0 to 1, despite this mechanical thrombectomy should not be withheld blindly for patients with moderate to severe disability, that is, mRS of 2 to 4. Our practice it to assess on a case-by-case basis and to confer with the patient's family.

NIHSS at Presentation

Most of the MT trials enrolled patients with NIHSS greater than or equal to 6, which is generally considered to be disabling. The efficacy of MT in patients with NIHSS less than 6 remains under investigation. Our practice is to offer MT based on the severity of deficits and resultant disability regardless of NIHSS, taking into account unique patient characteristics, for example, an isolated homonymous hemianopsia would result in an NIHSS of 2 but this deficit in a young aircraft pilot would be a career ending deficit but may not affect the life of an octogenarian as severely.

Location of the Large Vessel Occlusion in the Anterior Circulation

In the anterior circulation, most of the clinical trials included patients with ICA and proximal MCA trunk (M1) occlusion (Fig. 2). Patients with more distal MCA trunk or MCA branch occlusions (first-order branches in the Sylvian fissure are referred to as M2 segments) or occlusions of other vessels such as the ACA were either excluded or underrepresented. Hence the data available for safety and efficacy are applicable to distal ICA or proximal MCA LVO. The current AHA/ASA guidelines recommend limiting treatment to those vessels only. Pooled data from multiple series of MT patients with M2 occlusions have revealed generally good functional outcomes with reperfusion (mRS 0–1; OR 2.2, 95% confidence interval [CI] 1.0–4.7).[21]

Table 1
Modified Rankin Scale (mRS)
0 No symptoms
1 No significant disability despite symptoms. Able to carry out all usual activities and duties
2 Slight disability, unable to carry out all previous activities but able to look after own affairs without assistance
3 Moderate disability, requiring some help but able to walk without assistance
4 Moderately severe disability; unable to walk and attend to bodily needs without assistance
5 Severe disability, bedridden, incontinent, and requiring constant nursing care and attention
6 Dead

The major concern is that more distal occlusions tend to involve smaller vessels (<2 mm), which are associated with lower NIHSS scores and which are also more angulated, all of which may be associated with higher risks of ICH and lower net benefit. Our practice for LVO involving the distal M1, M2 branches, and the proximal ACA segments is to assess patients on a case-by-case basis and to offer MT only if deficits are disabling and the occlusion can be reached safely using available equipment.

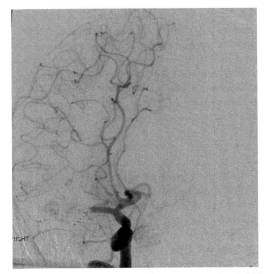

Fig. 2. Arrow points to right MCA proximal M1 segment occlusion.

Presentation 6 Hours or Less from Last Known Well (Early Window)

Six clinical trials published in 2015 compared MT with stent retrievers with intravenous rtPA alone or best medical therapy. These trials established the superiority of MT in patients presenting within 6 hours with a number needed to treat (NNT) to achieve functional independence ranging from 3 in the EXTEND-IA[22] trial to NNT of 7.5 in MR CLEAN trial.[23] A pooled meta-analysis of 5 of the clinical trials was performed by the HERMES collaboration and revealed an NNT of 2.6 to reduce disability by at least 1 grade on mRS. Patient's eligibility for MT mainly depends on the Alberta Stroke Program Early CT Score (ASPECTS). This is a 10-point score of the extent of infarction in the MCA territory on axial CT head or diffusion-weighted MRI. A score of 10 indicates no signs of early ischemia in the MCA territory, whereas a score of 0 indicates complete MCA early ischemic changes. Good outcome with mechanical thrombectomy was seen in patients with ASPECTS of greater than or equal to 6. Patients with ASPECTS less than 6 have less benefit and increased risk from mechanical thrombectomy, although it is not clear that the benefit of MT in low ASPECTS patients is not clinically meaningful. It is important that the ASPECTS be considered in the overall clinical context with the age of the patient, baseline level of independence, and patient/family preferences regarding goals of care in the setting of certain disability.

Presentation 6 to 24 Hours from Last Known Well (Late Window)

The AHA/ASA time window recommendations for MT were expanded to 16 hours after the results of the DEFUSE trial were published[24] and to 24 hours after the results of the DAWN[25] trial were published. Both DEFFUSE and DAWN selected patients for MT by using advanced imaging with CTP or MR perfusion. Both trials used the concept of infarct core (IC) to penumbra mismatch on perfusion imaging measured by automated software. Core infarct was defined equally in both trials as cerebral blood flow (CBF) less than 30% of the contralateral normal hemisphere CBF, whereas the penumbra was defined by a Tmax greater than 6 seconds, which is a region of reduced perfusion that was not yet included in the infarct core (Fig. 3).

DEFFUSE 3 enrolled patients up to 90 years of age with NIHSS greater than or equal to 6 and presenting within 6 to 16 hours of last known well. The trial required that the IC volume be less than 70 mL and an IC:penumbra

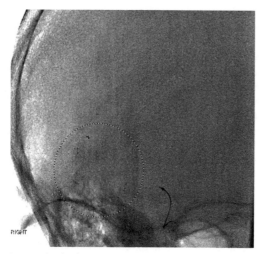

Fig. 3. Circle showing stent retriever deployed in the right middle cerebral artery.

mismatch of greater than 1.8. The trial was stopped early after enrollment of 182 patients due to efficacy of the treatment arm. Functional independence defined as mRS of 0 to 2 at 90 days was achieved in 44.6% in the mechanical thrombectomy arm compared with 16.7% in the medical treatment arm with ($P < .001$). The number NNT to achieve functional independence was 3.6.

The DAWN trial enrolled 206 patients between 6 and 24 hours from stroke onset with a more complex clinical and radiographic mismatch criteria. Penumbra was not directly assessed but was inferred based on clinical:IC mismatch: patients were categorized into 3 groups:

Group A: patients aged 80 years and older with NIHSS greater than or equal to 10 and infarct volume less than 21 mL.

Group B: patients younger than 80 years with NIHSS greater than or equal to 10 and infarct volume less than 31 mL.

Group C: patients younger than 80 years with NIHSS greater than or equal to 20 and infarct volume 31 to 51 mL.

Functional independence defined as mRS of 0 to 2 at 90 days was achieved in 49% in the MT arm compared with 13% in the medical arm. The NNT was 3. The rate of symptomatic ICH was not significantly different (6% with MT vs 3% with medical treatment, $P = .5$). These 2 trials have significantly changed the paradigm of acute stroke management in the late window. Mechanical thrombectomy outside the strict criteria set by DEFFUSE 3 and DAWN trials in the late window is considered experimental.

Furthermore, some have questioned the need for such strict imaging criteria, which can delay and restrict the number of patients treated; to address this issue there are several RCTs that are assessing the benefit of MT in patients with larger IC or ASPECT less than 6.

POSTERIOR CIRCULATION LARGE VESSEL OCCLUSION

The incidence of LVO in the posterior circulation including the VA, BA, or posterior cerebral arteries is much lower than in the anterior circulation. On the other hand, acute BA occlusion carries a higher risk of severe neurologic deficit and death. The randomized trials of MT did not include this patient population and as such the AHA/ASA guidelines did not support MT with the same level of vigor as in the anterior circulation. Recently the first international RCT comparing MT with standard medical treatment in BA occlusion (BASICS) was completed with disappointing results. MT performed within 6 hours of stroke onset showed no significant benefit compared with standard medical therapy for 90-day disability. However, the confidence intervals were very wide due to underrecruitment, and a substantial benefit of mechanical thrombectomy cannot be excluded based on this trial. On subgroup analysis there was a signal of benefit with MT for patients presenting with an NIHSS greater than or equal to 10.[26] The optimal patient selection and time window for mechanical thrombectomy in BA occlusion remain unclear. One of the major challenges is that imaging of the neural structures of the posterior circulation is limited by bony artifacts with conventional CT. MRI is far superior for the detection of acute ischemia but is time-consuming and may not be readily available. Another limitation of posterior circulation MT trials is that there is a higher prevalence of atherosclerotic occlusion as the cause of the LVO compared with anterior circulation trials that may be associated with less desirable angiographic outcomes and a higher rate of reocclusion with MT performed without angioplasty and stenting. Our current practice is to offer MT to patients with significant disability or NIHSS greater than 10 who do not have evidence of extensive pontine, midbrain, or thalamic infarction. If possible, we will perform a limited MRI, so called "wake-up MRI protocol," for patients presenting beyond 6 hours to rule out irreversible infarction of the brain stem before revascularization. Further studies with larger number of subjects are needed.

REPERFUSION AND FIRST PASS EFFECT

The main goal in acute stroke treatment is to achieve complete reperfusion to the affected area of the brain as soon as possible. The modified Thrombolysis in Cerebral Infarction (mTICI) score (Table 2) is the most widely used score across all MT trials that quantify reperfusion angiographically. TICI score is proved to predict outcomes. TICI 2b and higher is considered adequate reperfusion that is associated with improved outcomes in most of the clinical trials, although more recently it is recognized that the goal of MT should be TICI 2c or 3. In some cases, multiple passes of the stent retriever are needed to achieve reperfusion, and this is associated with higher rates of complications and futility. Achievement of reperfusion after a single stent retriever pass is associated with significantly better outcomes and is known as the first pass effect. The usage of balloon guide catheters (BGC) during MT is associated with increased first pass effect.[27]

STENT RETRIEVER VERSUS SUCTION THROMBECTOMY (THE COMPASS TRIAL)

MT can be performed using second-generation stent retrievers, distal aspiration catheters, or both together. The COMPASS trial randomized 270 patients with anterior circulation LVO to MT using catheter aspiration (AKA contact aspiration) only or stent retriever as first-line treatment. There was no difference in good functional outcomes at 90 days between the 2 groups with similar recanalization rates, indicating noninferiority of aspiration thrombectomy. Achievement of TICI 3 within 45 minutes was better with aspiration technique (34% vs 23%, $P = .05$), and time to groin puncture was shorter compared with patients treated with a stent retriever (25 minutes vs 35 minutes, $P = .03$).[28] However, a minority of the stent retriever procedures were performed with BGC catheters, which casts doubt on the validity of the comparison. There were no significant differences in rates of ICH, all-cause mortality, or overall safety. More recently the ASTER 2 trial conducted in France[29] showed that contact aspiration combined with a stent retriever had similar rates of TICI 2c/3 and clinical outcomes to stent retrievers with BGC catheter. The current AHA/ASA guidelines acknowledge noninferiority of contact aspiration. Our approach is to use stent retrievers and BGC catheters as first-line treatment except in cases of severe cervical tortuosity, dissection, or stenosis that may

preclude distal placement of the BGC, in which case we use contact aspiration along with a stent retriever.

GENERAL ANESTHESIA VERSUS CONSCIOUS SEDATION

Mechanical thrombectomy can be performed under general anesthesia (GA) or conscious sedation (CS). Several retrospective studies have shown that CS may be associated with better outcomes and lower mortality than GA.[30,31] Although GA leads to better control over patient movements, making it more comfortable for both patient and operator, it may add to the time of procedure initiation, carries the risk of significantly dropping blood pressure during induction, and masks the pain response associated with cerebral vessel stretching, vasospasm, and injury. On the other hand, CS may be associated with a higher risk of aspiration in some patients. Three small sample size randomized single-center trials (AnSTROKE, SIESTA, and GOLIATH) have shown noninferiority of GA compared with CS in clinical outcomes.[32–34] Because of the discrepancy between the very large retrospective analyses and the smaller RCTs, larger RCTs are being conducted. Until further conclusive evidence is available, we recommend individualizing anesthesia choice based on a patient's status. GA is preferred for severely agitated patients or those who are comatose and unable to maintain their airway. It is critical that drops in blood pressure be avoided during induction and maintenance of GA or CS.

Table 2	
Modified thrombolysis in cerebral infarction (mTICI) score	
mTICI 0	No recanalization
mTICI 1	Minimal recanalization
mTICI 2a	Partial recanalization and perfusion of < 50% of the vessel territory
mTICI 2b	Partial recanalization perfusion of > 50% of the vessel territory
mTICI 2c	Near-complete perfusion except for slow flow in a few distal cortical vessels or presence of small distal cortical emboli
mTICI 3	Complete reperfusion

BLOOD PRESSURE MANAGEMENT POSTMECHANICAL THROMBECTOMY

Hypertension is a well-known physiologic response to brain ischemia as part of cerebral autoregulation, which can maximize CBF via collaterals despite LVO. Blood pressure (BP) goals before and during MT should be to maintain BP at baseline unless it is very high (systolic BP > 220 mm Hg) or low (<130 mm Hg). BP goals after MT have been a topic of controversy. Good evidence data from RCTs are not yet available. The best available evidence comes from a multicenter retrospective study showing a higher likelihood of good outcome and lower odds of hemicraniectomy in the group of patients with systolic blood pressure less than 140 mm Hg after successful recanalization.[35] Very elevated BP after MT has been associated with poor outcomes but so has very low BP resulting in a U-shaped curve.[36,37] Higher SBP targets can be considered on a case-by-case basis in patients who achieve partial recanalization in order to maintain perfusion to the tissue at risk. Regardless of BP goal, close observation in dedicated stroke units or neurologic critical care units by dedicated nurses and physicians is essential and has been associated with improved neurologic outcomes.[38]

DISCLOSURE

O. Alsrouji has nothing to disclose. A. Chebl has received (minor) honoraria for consulting work from Medtronic Inc, Cerenovus Inc.

REFERENCE

1. Lakomkin N, Dhamoon M, Carroll K, et al. Prevalence of large vessel occlusion in patients presenting with acute ischemic stroke: a 10-year systematic review of the literature. J Neurointerv Surg 2019; 11(3):241–5.

2. Saver JL. Time is brain–quantified. Stroke 2006; 37(1):263–6.

3. Beume LA, Hieber M, Kaller CP, et al. Large Vessel Occlusion in Acute Stroke. Stroke 2018;49(10): 2323–9.

4. Heldner MR, Hsieh K, Broeg-Morvay A, et al. Clinical prediction of large vessel occlusion in anterior circulation stroke: mission impossible? J Neurol 2016;263(8):1633–40.

5. Mayer SA, Viarasilpa T, Panyavachiraporn N, et al. CTA-for-all: impact of emergency computed tomographic angiography for all patients with stroke presenting within 24 hours of onset. Stroke 2020; 51(1):331–4.

6. Saqqur M, Uchino K, Demchuk AM, et al. Site of arterial occlusion identified by transcranial Doppler predicts the response to intravenous thrombolysis for stroke. Stroke 2007;38(3):948–54.

7. Linfante I, Llinas RH, Selim M, et al. Clinical and vascular outcome in internal carotid artery versus middle cerebral artery occlusions after intravenous tissue plasminogen activator. Stroke 2002;33(8): 2066–71.

8. Yoo J, Baek JH, Park H, et al. Thrombus volume as a predictor of nonrecanalization after intravenous thrombolysis in acute stroke. Stroke 2018;49(9): 2108–15.

9. Yang P, Zhang Y, Zhang L, et al. Endovascular thrombectomy with or without intravenous alteplase in acute stroke. N Engl J Med 2020;382(21): 1981–93.

10. Suzuki K, Matsumaru Y, Takeuchi M, et al. Effect of mechanical thrombectomy without vs with intravenous thrombolysis on functional outcome among patients with acute ischemic stroke: the SKIP randomized clinical trial. JAMA 2021;325(3):244–53.

11. Wang Y, Wu X, Zhu C, et al. Bridging thrombolysis achieved better outcomes than direct thrombectomy after large vessel occlusion: an updated meta-analysis. Stroke 2021;52(1):356–65.

12. Powers WJ, Rabinstein AA, Ackerson T, et al. Guidelines for the early management of patients with acute ischemic stroke: 2019 update to the 2018 guidelines for the early management of acute ischemic stroke: a guideline for healthcare professionals from the american heart association/american stroke association. Stroke 2019;50(12):e344–418 [published correction appears in stroke. 2019 Dec;50(12):e440-e441].

13. Katsanos AH, Safouris A, Sarraj A, et al. Intravenous thrombolysis with tenecteplase in patients with large vessel occlusions: systematic review and meta-analysis. Stroke 2021;52(1):308–12.

14. Broderick JP, Palesch YY, Demchuk AM, et al. Endovascular therapy after intravenous t-PA versus t-PA alone for stroke. N Engl J Med 2013;368(10): 893–903.

15. Kidwell CS, Jahan R, Gornbein J, et al. A trial of imaging selection and endovascular treatment for ischemic stroke. N Engl J Med 2013;368(10):914–23.

16. Ciccone A, Valvassori L, Nichelatti M, et al. Endovascular treatment for acute ischemic stroke. N Engl J Med 2013;368(10):904–13.

17. Bhatia K, Kortman H, Blair C, et al. Mechanical thrombectomy in pediatric stroke: systematic review, individual patient data meta-analysis, and case series. J Neurosurg Pediatr 2019;1–14. https://doi.org/10.3171/2019.5.PEDS19126.

18. Al-Mufti F, Schirmer CM, Starke RM, et al. Thrombectomy in special populations: report of the Society of NeuroInterventional Surgery Standards and

Guidelines Committee [published online ahead of print, 2021 Jul 8]. J Neurointerv Surg 2021. https://doi.org/10.1136/neurintsurg-2021-017888.

19. Seker F, Pfaff J, Schönenberger S, et al. Clinical outcome after thrombectomy in patients with stroke with premorbid modified rankin scale scores of 3 and 4: a cohort study with 136 patients. AJNR Am J Neuroradiol 2019;40(2):283–6.

20. Salwi S, Cutting S, Salgado AD, et al. Mechanical thrombectomy in patients with ischemic stroke with prestroke disability. Stroke 2020;51(5):1539–45.

21. Lemmens R, Hamilton SA, Liebeskind DS, et al. Effect of endovascular reperfusion in relation to site of arterial occlusion. Neurology 2016;86(8):762–70.

22. Campbell BC, Mitchell PJ, Kleinig TJ, et al. Endovascular therapy for ischemic stroke with perfusion-imaging selection. N Engl J Med 2015; 372(11):1009–18.

23. Berkhemer OA, Fransen PS, Beumer D, et al. A randomized trial of intraarterial treatment for acute ischemic stroke. N Engl J Med 2015;372(1): 11–20.

24. Albers GW, Marks MP, Kemp S, et al. Thrombectomy for stroke at 6 to 16 hours with selection by perfusion imaging. N Engl J Med 2018;378(8): 708–18.

25. Nogueira RG, Jadhav AP, Haussen DC, et al. Thrombectomy 6 to 24 hours after stroke with a mismatch between deficit and infarct. N Engl J Med 2018;378(1):11–21.

26. Langezaal LCM, van der Hoeven EJRJ, Mont'Alverne FJA, et al. Endovascular therapy for stroke due to basilar-artery occlusion. N Engl J Med 2021;384(20):1910–20.

27. Zaidat OO, Castonguay AC, Linfante I, et al. First Pass Effect: A New Measure for Stroke Thrombectomy Devices. Stroke 2018;49(3):660–6. https://doi.org/10.1161/STROKEAHA.117.020315.

28. Turk AS 3rd, Siddiqui A, Fifi JT, et al. Aspiration thrombectomy versus stent retriever thrombectomy as first-line approach for large vessel occlusion (COMPASS): a multicentre, randomised, open label, blinded outcome, non-inferiority trial. Lancet 2019;393(10175):998–1008.

29. Lapergue B, Blanc R, Costalat V, et al. Effect of thrombectomy with combined contact aspiration and stent retriever vs stent retriever alone on revascularization in patients with acute ischemic stroke and large vessel occlusion: the ASTER2 randomized clinical trial. JAMA 2021;326(12):1158–69.

30. Abou-Chebl A, Lin R, Hussain MS, et al. Conscious sedation versus general anesthesia during endovascular therapy for acute anterior circulation stroke: preliminary results from a retrospective, multicenter study. Stroke 2010;41(6):1175–9.

31. Wan TF, Xu R, Zhao ZA, et al. Outcomes of general anesthesia versus conscious sedation for Stroke undergoing endovascular treatment: a meta-analysis. BMC Anesthesiol 2019;19(1):69.

32. Löwhagen Hendén P, Rentzos A, Karlsson JE, et al. General anesthesia versus conscious sedation for endovascular treatment of acute ischemic stroke: the anstroke trial (anesthesia during stroke). Stroke 2017;48(6):1601–7.

33. Schönenberger S, Möhlenbruch M, Pfaff J, et al. Sedation vs. intubation for endovascular stroke treatment (SIESTA) - a randomized monocentric trial. Int J Stroke 2015;10(6):969–78.

34. Simonsen CZ, Yoo AJ, Sørensen LH, et al. Effect of general anesthesia and conscious sedation during endovascular therapy on infarct growth and clinical outcomes in acute ischemic stroke: a randomized clinical trial. JAMA Neurol 2018;75(4):470–7.

35. Anadani M, Arthur AS, Tsivgoulis G, et al. Blood pressure goals and clinical outcomes after successful endovascular therapy: a multicenter study. Ann Neurol 2020;87(6):830–9.

36. Malhotra K, Goyal N, Katsanos AH, et al. Association of blood pressure with outcomes in acute stroke thrombectomy. Hypertension 2020;75(3): 730–9.

37. Vemmos KN, Tsivgoulis G, Spengos K, et al. U-shaped relationship between mortality and admission blood pressure in patients with acute stroke. J Intern Med 2004;255(2):257–65.

38. How do stroke units improve patient outcomes? A collaborative systematic review of the randomized trials. Stroke 1997;28(11):2139–44.

Percutaneous Large Thrombus and Vegetation Evacuation in the Catheterization Laboratory

Madhan Shanmugasundaram, MD*,
Arka Chatterjee, MD, Kwan Lee, MD

KEYWORDS

- AngioVac • Vacuum aspiration thrombectomy • Extracorporeal membrane oxygenation
- Tricuspid valve endocarditis • Cardiac implantable electronic devices • Iliocaval thrombus
- Right atrial mass

KEY POINTS

- The presence of right heart or iliocaval thrombi in patients with pulmonary embolism is associated with a high mortality risk.
- The AngioVac percutaneous vacuum-assisted thrombectomy device is a treatment option for patients with iliocaval or right heart thrombi who are at high surgical risk or poor candidates for thrombolytic therapy.
- Tricuspid valve endocarditis accounts for ~10% of all endocarditis and surgery is associated with high morbidity and mortality including recurrent infections in the prosthetic valve.
- The safety of the AngioVac system to debulk tricuspid and cardiac implantable electronic device vegetations has been well established and may have a role in these patients.
- Because of its bulky nature and reports of right ventricular perforation, use of the AngioVac thrombectomy system is generally not recommended for pulmonary embolism.

INTRODUCTION

Intracardiac masses are not an uncommon clinical problem in current day cardiovascular practice. These include thrombi, vegetations, or tumors.[1,2] Symptomsrange from intracardiac obstruction, arrhythmias, stroke, or systemic embolism. Historically intracardiac masses have been underdiagnosed and often noticed postmortem, but with the advances in cardiovascular imaging, these masses have been increasingly diagnosed in contemporary practice. In addition to intracardiac masses, large intravascular thrombi of the iliocaval system are associated with an increased risk of pulmonary embolism (PE). Right heart thrombi are only seen in approximately 4% of all patients with PE but they are associated with high mortality and morbidity if untreated.[3,4] Right-sided infective endocarditis (IE) accounts for 5% to 10% of all IE cases and is typically associated with intravenous drug use, intracardiac devices, and central venous catheters. If left untreated right-sided IE is associated with high morbidity because of valve regurgitation or septic PE. The management of intracardiac thrombi or intravascular thrombi is determined by the underlying cause, location, and presence of comorbidities but surgery remains the gold standard approach. Most patients with right-sided IE undergo surgery.[5] However, some of these patients have high surgical risk because of the presence of

Section of Cardiology, Department of Internal Medicine, Banner University Medical Center, Sarver Heart Center, 1501 North Campbell Avenue, Tucson, AZ 85724, USA
* Corresponding author.
E-mail address: msundaram@shc.arizona.edu

Intervent Cardiol Clin 11 (2022) 349–358
https://doi.org/10.1016/j.iccl.2022.03.007
2211-7458/22/© 2022 Elsevier Inc. All rights reserved.

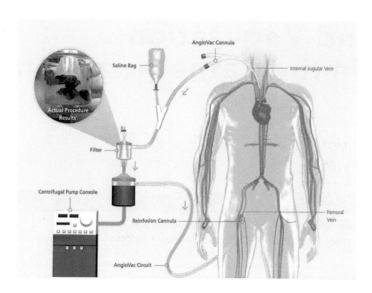

Fig. 1. AngioVac system. (Reproduced with permission from Basman et al: J Card Surg. 2018;33:666–672.[47])

comorbidities. Recent advancements in catheter-based technologies have expanded percutaneous options for treatment of these large thrombi or vegetation in high-surgical-risk patients. For thrombi, management includes anticoagulation alone or combined with thrombolytic therapy, which is either systemically administered or catheter directed.[6–8] There is lack of consensus when it comes to the management of right heart thrombus. Surgical embolectomy and thrombolytic therapy have been described in the literature.[9] Percutaneous options may be preferred in some patients depending on the complexity of the disease process, comorbidities, bleeding, and surgical risk. Percutaneous aspiration thrombectomy/vacuum-assisted thrombectomy may benefit patients with concurrent PE or to prevent significant PE who have extensive iliocaval thrombus or intracardiac mass in transit who are poor candidates for thrombolytic therapy or surgical embolectomy. The AngioVac system (Angiodynamics, Latham, NY) is the most used device for removal of intracardiac and intravascular materials[10] but the INARI FlowTriever (Inari Medical, Irvine, CA) and Penumbra mechanical thrombectomy systems (Penumbra, Alameda, CA) have also been used. The focus of this review is percutaneous large thrombus and vegetation management using the AngioVac system.

AngioVac SYSTEM

The AngioVac system consists of a 22F catheter outflow canula with a balloon-actuated, expandable funnel-shaped distal tip that requires a 26F catheter introducer system. The most used 26F catheter sheath is a Gore DrySeal (W.L. Gore & Associates Inc, Flagstaff, AZ) sheath that is placed percutaneously or via surgical cut down. The outflow canula is connected to a filter (to remove the intravascular or intracardiac debris) and a centrifugal pump head that generates up to 80 mm Hg negative suction pressure. The filtered blood is then returned to the body via a 16F catheter inflow canula as shown in Fig. 1. The large luminal diameter of the system ensures en bloc removal of large thrombi and vegetation with lower risk of fragmentation or embolization. The AngioVac system was Food and Drug Administration approved in 2009 for the removal of unwanted intravascular materials including thrombus, tumor, and foreign bodies via a venovenous extracorporeal membranous oxygenation (ECMO) circuit. Since its approval there have been several reports of this system being used for off-label indications, such as debulking or removal of intracardiac masses including thrombus, tricuspid valve vegetations, and catheter-related thrombi or vegetations. The current generation of the system is available with either a 20-degree or a 180-degree angled tip, which enables easier navigation depending on the indication. The tip is radiopaque, which facilitates fluoroscopic guidance during the procedure and the funnel tip prevents clogging of the canula and reduces embolization. The canula itself is supported by kink-resistant stainless steel coiled wire within the body. The funnel tip is self-expanding and needs to be unsheathed from the delivery sheath once in the superior vena cava (SVC) or right atrium

(RA). This sliding sheath controls the position and helps form the curve of the canula, also helping with steering and control. There is a Y-adaptor with Tuohy insert that is connected to the outflow canula, which allows for introduction of 0.035-inch guidewire through the side port or catheter if needed.

AngioVac PROCEDURE AND SETUP

The procedure is typically performed under general anesthesia, although it can be done under conscious sedation. Imaging guidance is provided by transesophageal echocardiogram (TEE) or intracardiac echocardiogram. Cardiac anesthesiologists and perfusionists are critical members of the team during these procedures. Depending on the indication, the outflow canula is placed in the internal jugular (IJ) or common femoral vein. For SVC and iliocaval thrombectomies femoral venous access is preferred. For RA thrombus, tricuspid vegetation, or PE, right IJ access is used. The inflow canula is almost always positioned in the femoral vein. After obtaining access, serial dilations are typically performed over a 0.035-inch stiff wire before placing a 26Fr Gore DrySeal sheath for the outflow canula. The size of the inflow canula can vary from 16 to 19Fr and is placed in a similar fashion. During this time, the ECMO circuit is deaired and primed using the priming solution and is clamped. After placing the large-bore sheaths, intravenous heparin is administered for a target activated clotting time of 250 to 300 seconds. Following this the venovenous ECMO circuit is established. After this the AngioVac canula is advanced under fluoroscopic and TEE guidance to the target area and the ECMO circuit flow is slowly increased up to 5 L/min. Once aspiration is satisfactorily completed, hemostasis is achieved using a figure-of-eight or purse string sutures. Alternatively, two Perclose ProGlide suture devices (Abbott Vascular, Chicago, IL) used in a "preclose" fashion have been reported.

CLINICAL APPLICATIONS
Right Heart Thrombi and Iliocaval Thrombi
Right heart, specifically right atrial thrombi, typically arise from iliocaval system but rarely could be from upper extremity veins or associated with central venous catheters. They can migrate to the pulmonary arteries causing PE or across a patent foramen ovale causing systemic embolism or stroke. The presence of right heart thrombi in patients with PE confers a high risk of mortality and warrants removal either surgically or percutaneously.[11] Thrombolytics and

anticoagulants have been shown to be beneficial but are associated with significant bleeding risk including intracranial bleeding.[12] There have been several case reports and series that demonstrate technical success with the AngioVac system for removal of right heart thrombi and iliocaval thrombi with lower rates of complications. Acute thrombi are more likely to be aspirated with high technical success compared with chronic thrombi.[13]

Al Badri and colleagues[11] published their experience of RA thrombus aspiration in six patients using the AngioVac system. This case series demonstrated high technical success rate with no major complications including periprocedural bleeding. Resnik and colleagues[14] published their early experience in a single-center case series where they included seven consecutive critically ill patients with RA/iliac vein or vena caval thrombi who underwent thrombus aspiration. They showed complete thrombus aspiration in all patients and one distal embolization with no other major complications. Another case series included 16 consecutive patients, most of whom had RA or iliocaval thrombi and underwent successful thrombus aspiration using the AngioVac system with no periprocedural mortality. The only major complication in this series of patients was acute blood loss anemia requiring transfusion.[15] There have been reported cases of successful AngioVac thrombectomy of RA thrombi in patients who were poor thrombolytic or surgical candidates.[16,17]

Salsamendi and colleagues[18] reported their experience with the AngioVac system in seven patients with intracardiac or intravascular thrombi, including one patient with thrombi in the Fontan circuit. They demonstrated the efficacy and safety of this system in their series and noted they had partial success in the aspiration of chronic thrombi.

The AngioVac system has a higher success rate with complete thrombus aspiration in the iliocaval system. Smith and colleagues[10] reported three cases of successful aspiration in patients with iliocaval thrombi who failed anticoagulant therapy. The largest case series of thrombus aspiration included 15 patients, most of whom had RA thrombus with a greater than 70% success rate.[19] Table 1 summarizes all published case series of vacuum-assisted thrombectomy in patients with RA or iliac thrombi. The Registry of AngioVac Procedures in Detail (RAPID) Study is a multicenter prospective registry of AngioVac procedures for different indications. It is the largest published series to date, including 234 patients, most

Table 1
Case series of AngioVac system in RA/iliocaval thrombi

Case Series	Number of Patients	Location of Thrombus (Number of Patients)
Donaldson et al,[19] 2015	15	RA (11) Iliocaval (4)
D'Ayala et al,[13] 2017	9	RA (5) Iliocaval (4)
Al Badri et al,[11] 2016	7	RA (7)
Resnick et al,[14] 2016	7	RA (4) Iliocaval (3)
Salsamendi et al,[18] 2015	5	RA (1) Iliocaval (4)
Smith et al,[10] 2014	3	Iliocaval (3)

(>70%) of which had iliocaval thrombi. This series established the safety and efficacy of the AngioVac system in real-world practice. Less than 1% procedure-related death was reported, with vascular trauma and major bleeding the most common complications in this large database.[20]

Pulmonary Embolism

There have been limited cases published examining the use of the AngioVac system in patients with PE. This may be due to the the the bulky nature of the system and inability to successfully and safely traverse the right heart to reach the pulmonary artery. Because of the large-caliber nature of this system, it can only be used for saddle or main pulmonary artery emboli. Al Hakim and colleagues reported a series of five patients with PE, of which four of them were massive and one submassive on presentation who underwent AngioVac pulmonary thrombectomy.[21] The patients had either a contraindication to lytic therapy or were too sick for surgery. Two of these cases were successful and one patient had right ventricular free wall perforation because of the AngioVac canula. Four of these patients died within 7 days indicating a sick cohort. The technique the operators used included placing the AngioVac canula in the main pulmonary artery, after which they inflated a balloon in the thrombus distally to cause fragmentation. Following this, the inflated balloon was pulled back to drag the thrombi closer to the canula. Another case series demonstrated a low success rate (~30%) for patients

with PE using the AngioVac system.[13] There is not enough evidence to support the routine use of AngioVac thrombectomy for patients with PE.

Infective Endocarditis

Antibiotic therapy is critical for the management of tricuspid endocarditis but patients with large vegetation, persistent bacteremia, fungal infection, or septic embolization need surgery.[22,23] Surgery has its drawbacks in these patients including 5% to 10% mortality risk, surgical morbidity, and recurrent infection of prosthetic valves.[24,25] AngioVac debulking of tricuspid valve (TV) vegetation has been well described now and is considered in patients with high surgical risk as a bridge to surgery. A retrospective single-center case series of 33 patients with TV endocarditis who underwent AngioVac debulking demonstrated safety and efficacy in these patients. They defined satisfactory debulking as greater than 1 cm removal of particulate material or the inability to remove any additional material. The outflow canula was placed in the right IJ and the inflow canula was placed in the common femoral vein with conscious sedation and TEE guidance in all procedures. The authors reported a significant reduction in the size of the TV vegetation during follow-up echocardiography. There were no procedure-related deaths, but there was a 9% death rate during the index hospitalization and a 9% risk of needing TV surgery for severe tricuspid regurgitation post-AngioVac. Hence, the authors concluded that AngioVac debulking seems to be a safe alternative to surgery in high-surgical-risk patients with TV endocarditis.[26] There have been several other case reports demonstrating feasibility, efficacy in debulking, and safety of the AngioVac system in patients with TV endocarditis.[27–31] Fig. 2 shows a case of successful AngioVac debulking of a vegetation from a bioprosthetic tricuspid valve (patient deemed high surgical risk).

Cardiac Implantable Electronic Devices

Over the last decade the implantation of cardiac implantable electronic devices (CIEDs; pacemakers, implantable cardioverter defibrillators, and cardiac resynchronization therapies) has increased exponentially following their positive impact on morbidity and mortality. There has also been an increasing trend in CIED infections with estimates ranging between 0.1% and almost 20%.[32,33] More contemporary studies show infection rates of almost 6%.[34] Regardless, CIED infections are associated with significant

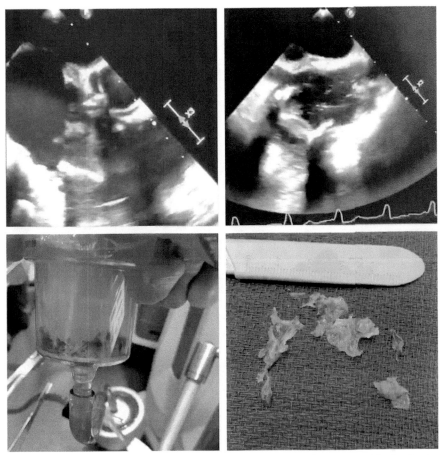

Fig. 2. Case of successful AngioVac debulking of vegetation from bioprosthetic tricuspid valve (patient deemed high surgical risk).

morbidity and mortality. Device infections can either be superficial (involving the pocket or generator) or deep (involving intracardiac/intravascular leads). Heart Rhythm Society consensus guidelines recommend antibiotic therapy and infected device removal.[35] Larger lead infections have more embolization risk during extraction and thus are referred for surgical removal occasionally, but these patients are generally a higher risk cohort. The AngioVac system has been successfully used to debulk large lead vegetations before extraction to minimize embolization risk. A recently published large case series included 20 patients with CIED vegetation with sizes ranging between 2 and 6 cm who underwent AngioVac removal of lead vegetation followed by lead extraction. This study demonstrated feasibility, efficacy in removal of lead vegetation using the AngioVac system with no safety signal. No major procedural complications were seen in this series.[36] Patel and colleagues[37] demonstrated safety and efficacy

of the AngioVac system in their case series of three patients with large (>2 cm) lead vegetation who were high surgical risk. Similarly Godara and colleagues[38] published their single-center experience of AngioVac-mediated removal of large lead vegetations (>2 cm) in eight patients where they demonstrated feasibility and safety. Based on these studies it seems reasonable to consider AngioVac-mediated debulking of large lead vegetation (>2 cm) before lead extraction to minimize embolic risk. Fig. 3 shows a patient with an infected pacemaker lead who underwent lead extraction, after which the vegetation sheared off from the lead and stuck to the RA/SVC junction. This was successfully retrieved later using an AngioVac device before reimplanting a new device.

Miscellaneous
Primary cardiac tumors are rare but most of them tend to be metastatic. There have been case reports of an AngioVac used to remove

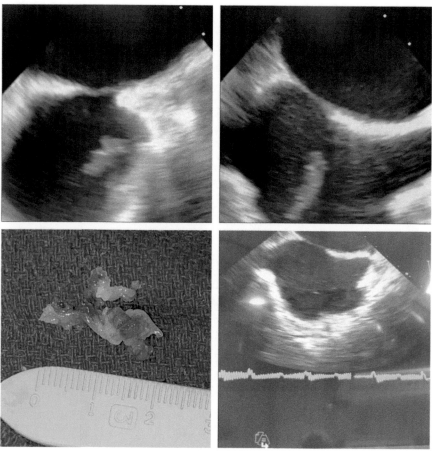

Fig. 3. Patient with infected pacemaker lead who underwent lead extraction and the vegetation sheared off from the lead and stuck to the RA/SVC junction, which was successfully retrieved later using AngioVac device.

intracardiac tumors. Joseph-Alexis and colleagues[39] demonstrated successful removal of a pulmonary valve papillary fibroelastoma using an AngioVac system. Bhagat and colleagues[40] published their experience of removal of right atrial papillary fibroelastoma using AngioVac system. There have been few case reports describing the use of an AngioVac system for removal of intravascular thrombi from the aorta. Quintar and colleagues[41] reported a case of ascending aortic large thrombus removal using an AngioVac system in a patient who presented with recurrent stroke. They achieved access to the aorta by transcaval access to place the outflow canula and the inflow canula was placed in the contralateral femoral vein. Bilateral Sentinel cerebral protection device (Boston Scientific, Marlborough, MA) was used in this patient and authors reported successful removal of the arch thrombus under TEE and fluoroscopic guidance without any major

complications. Another case of a patient presenting with acute mesenteric ischemia and abdominal aortic thrombi not responding to intravenous anticoagulation was treated using an AngioVac system. Here the outflow canula was placed via right femoral artery using surgical cut down and the inflow canula was placed via the femoral vein.[42] Kang and colleagues[43] reported removal of distal thoracic aortic thrombi in a patient with angiosarcoma who presented with acute limb ischemia and emboli to the spleen and lower extremities. In this patient the authors placed the 26F catheter sheath and outflow canula via the right common femoral artery, accessed percutaneously and closed at the end using Perclose Proglide closure devices. Frisoli and colleagues[44] reported a patient who presented with an acute stroke and was found to have a large ascending aortic thrombus, which was successfully removed using the AngioVac system via the right common femoral artery approach. Given the location of this thrombus the authors placed a Sentinel cerebral protection system via the right radial approach and balloon occluded the left subclavian artery via left radial access to avoid distal embolization. Tsilimparis and colleagues[45] reported their experience of removal of a large ascending aortic thrombus using the AngioVac system in a patient with metastatic lung cancer who was deemed to be a poor surgical candidate. They used left subclavian arterial access via surgical cut down for this patient. AngioVac has also been used to debulk left atrial masses/thrombus with a transseptal approach as reported by Ashukem and colleagues[46] in a patient with obstructive shock after a transcatheter mitral valve replacement. Box 1 outlines common indications for the AngioVac.

COMPLICATIONS

Despite its benefits and efficacy, the AngioVac system is associated with complications, which need to be reviewed before considering this system. These include vascular access site complications needing further therapy; bleeding requiring blood transfusion; and distal embolization that, if occurring in the pulmonary system, may cause sudden cardiopulmonary collapse. Right heart perforation has been described in cases where this system was used for PE aspiration. Rare instances of procedure-related deaths have been reported. In the largest prospective, multicenter registry of 234 patients who underwent AngioVac procedure, death occurred in less than 1% of patients, whereas bleeding (~4%) and vascular injury (3.5%) occurred more commonly.[20] Box 2 lists some common complications reported with AngioVac.

SUMMARY

The AngioVac system seems to be a safe alternative percutaneous strategy to remove intracardiac or intravascular thrombi and to debulk tricuspid valve or CIED vegetations in high-surgical-risk patients. The success rate for removal of iliocaval and RA thrombi is high with the AngioVac system making this device a much-needed addition to the interventionalist's toolbox. The rigid and bulky nature of this system makes it a less attractive option for percutaneous pulmonary embolectomy at this time, especially given reports of right heart perforation in some cases. Large-bore access management skills and use of ECMO are critical for the successful use of this system.

CLINICS CARE POINTS

- Iliocaval and right heart thrombi are not uncommon. They are associated with a high risk of mortality in patients with pulmonary embolism.

- Although surgery remains the gold standard treatment of intravascular and intracardiac thrombi, it is not often feasible in these patients because of their comorbidities. Also, surgery is associated with high risk of morbidity and mortality.

- Percutaneous vacuum-assisted thrombectomy using the AngioVac system has been shown to be effective and safe in patients with high surgical risk.

- AngioVac uses a venovenous extracorporeal membrane oxygenation (ECMO) system where the outflow (AngioVac) canula is 22F catheter (introduced through 26F catheter sheath), connected via a filter (to remove debris) and inflow canula (16–19F catheter).

- Commonly used access sites include right internal jugular vein and right and left common femoral veins.

- Ultrasound-guided access is recommended to minimize access site vascular complications.

- After achieving access, the track is serially dilated over a stiff wire to facilitate smooth placement of the 26F catheter sheath (Gore DrySeal) or return canula.

- Intravenous heparin is used for anticoagulation before initiating ECMO circuit and is monitored via activated clotting time measurement (250–300 seconds).

- These cases are performed in collaboration with cardiac anesthesiologist and cardiac perfusion team.

- TEE is used for procedural imaging guidance, although intracardiac echocardiogram is also used.

- Hemostasis is achieved using skin sutures (purse string or figure-of-eight) or two Perclose Proglide sutures (preclose technique).

- Role of AngioVac in debulking of tricuspid valve vegetations and infections of cardiac implantable electronic devices (CIEDs) has been well published.

- AngioVac system is associated with increased risk of cardiac chamber perforation when used for pulmonary embolectomy, hence it is not recommended for patients with PE.

- Complications include procedure-related death (rare), chamber perforation (right ventricular perforation when used for PE), arrhythmias, bleeding (requiring transfusion), and vascular complication.

DISCLOSURE

None of the authors have any relevant financial conflicts of interest to disclose.

REFERENCES

1. Behrens G, Bjarnason H. Venous thromboembolic disease: the use of the aspiration thrombectomy device AngioVac. Semin Intervent Radiol 2015; 32(4):374–8.

2. Enezate TH, Kumar A, Aggarwal K, et al. Non-surgical extraction of right atrial mass by AngioVac aspiration device under fluoroscopic and transesophageal echocardiographic guidance. Cardiovasc Diagn Ther 2017;7(3):331–5.

3. Chartier L, Bera J, Delomez M, et al. Free-floating thrombi in the right heart: diagnosis, management, and prognostic indexes in 38 consecutive patients. Circulation 1999;99(21):2779–83.

4. Carson JL, Kelley MA, Duff A, et al. The clinical course of pulmonary embolism. N Engl J Med 1992;326(19):1240–5.

5. Chairs ASToIECGWC, Pettersson GB, Coselli JS, et al. 2016 The American Association for Thoracic Surgery (AATS) consensus guidelines: surgical treatment of infective endocarditis: executive summary. J Thorac Cardiovasc Surg 2017;153(6):1241–58.e9.

6. Vedantham S, Goldhaber SZ, Julian JA, et al. Pharmacomechanical catheter-directed thrombolysis for deep-vein thrombosis. N Engl J Med 2017; 377(23):2240–52.

7. Parikh S, Motarjeme A, McNamara T, et al. Ultrasound-accelerated thrombolysis for the treatment of deep vein thrombosis: initial clinical experience. J Vasc Interv Radiol 2008;19(4):521–8.

8. Kinney EL, Wright RJ. Efficacy of treatment of patients with echocardiographically detected right-sided heart thrombi: a meta-analysis. Am Heart J 1989;118(3):569–73.

9. Otoupalova E, Dalal B, Renard B. Right heart thrombus in transit: a series of two cases. Crit Ultrasound J 2017;9(1):14.

10. Smith SJ, Behrens G, Sewall LE, et al. Vacuum-assisted thrombectomy device (AngioVac) in the management of symptomatic iliocaval thrombosis. J Vasc Interv Radiol 2014;25(3):425–30.

11. Al Badri A, Kliger C, Weiss D, et al. Right atrial vacuum-assisted thrombectomy: single-center experience. J Invasive Cardiol 2016;28(5):196–201.

12. Rose PS, Punjabi NM, Pearse DB. Treatment of right heart thromboemboli. Chest 2002;121(3):806–14.

13. D'Ayala M, Worku B, Gulkarov I, et al. Factors associated with successful thrombus extraction with the AngioVac device: an institutional experience. Ann Vasc Surg 2017;38:242–7.

14. Resnick SA, O'Brien D, Strain D, et al. Single-center experience using AngioVac with extracorporeal bypass for mechanical thrombectomy of atrial and central vein thrombi. J Vasc Interv Radiol 2016;27(5):723–729 e721.

15. Rajput FA, Du L, Woods M, et al. Percutaneous vacuum-assisted thrombectomy using AngioVac aspiration system. Cardiovasc Revasc Med 2020;21(4):489–93.

16. Dudiy Y, Kronzon I, Cohen HA, et al. Vacuum thrombectomy of large right atrial thrombus. Catheter Cardiovasc Interv 2012;79(2):344–7.

17. Nickel B, McClure T, Moriarty J. A novel technique for endovascular removal of large volume right atrial tumor thrombus. Cardiovasc Intervent Radiol 2015;38(4):1021–4.

18. Salsamendi J, Doshi M, Bhatia S, et al. Single center experience with the AngioVac aspiration system. Cardiovasc Intervent Radiol 2015;38(4):998–1004.

19. Donaldson CW, Baker JN, Narayan RL, et al. Thrombectomy using suction filtration and venovenous bypass: single center experience with a novel device. Catheter Cardiovasc Interv 2015;86(2):E81–7.

20. Moriarty JM, Rueda V, Liao M, et al. Endovascular removal of thrombus and right heart masses using the AngioVac system: results of 234 patients from the prospective, multicenter Registry of AngioVac Procedures In Detail (RAPID). J Vasc Interv Radiol 2021;32(4):549–557 e543.

21. Al-Hakim R, Park J, Bansal A, et al. Early experience with AngioVac aspiration in the pulmonary arteries. J Vasc Interv Radiol 2016;27(5):730–4.

22. Robbins MJ, Frater RW, Soeiro R, et al. Influence of vegetation size on clinical outcome of right-sided infective endocarditis. Am J Med 1986;80(2):165–71.

23. Kang DH, Kim YJ, Kim SH, et al. Early surgery versus conventional treatment for infective endocarditis. N Engl J Med 2012;366(26):2466–73.

24. Gaca JG, Sheng S, Daneshmand M, et al. Current outcomes for tricuspid valve infective endocarditis surgery in North America. Ann Thorac Surg 2013;96(4):1374–81.

25. Thourani VH, Sarin EL, Kilgo PD, et al. Short- and long-term outcomes in patients undergoing valve surgery with end-stage renal failure receiving chronic hemodialysis. J Thorac Cardiovasc Surg 2012;144(1):117–23.

26. George B, Voelkel A, Kotter J, et al. A novel approach to percutaneous removal of large tricuspid valve vegetations using suction filtration and venovenous bypass: a single center experience. Catheter Cardiovasc Interv 2017;90(6):1009–15.

27. Bangalore S, Alviar CL, Vlahakis S, et al. Tricuspid valve vegetation debulking using the AngioVac system. Catheter Cardiovasc Interv 2021;98(3):E475–7.

28. Zern EK, Ramirez PR, Rubin J, et al. Severe tricuspid valve endocarditis: a tale of 2 circuits. JACC Case Rep 2021;3(11):1343–9.

29. Bisleri G, Hassan S, Wajid H, et al. Percutaneous aspiration of vegetation from tricuspid valve infective endocarditis. Multimed Man Cardiothorac Surg 2020;2020.

30. Wallenhorst P, Rutland J, Gurley J, et al. Use of AngioVac for removal of tricuspid valve vegetation. J Heart Valve Dis 2018;27(1):120–3.

31. Abubakar H, Rashed A, Subahi A, et al. AngioVac system used for vegetation debulking in a patient with tricuspid valve endocarditis: a case report and review of the literature. Case Rep Cardiol 2017;2017:1923505.

32. Conklin EF, Giannelli S Jr, Nealon TF Jr. Four hundred consecutive patients with permanent transvenous pacemakers. J Thorac Cardiovasc Surg 1975;69(1):1–7.

33. Bluhm G. Pacemaker infections. A clinical study with special reference to prophylactic use of some isoxazolyl penicillins. Acta Med Scand Suppl 1985;699:1–62.

34. Sridhar AR, Lavu M, Yarlagadda V, et al. Cardiac implantable electronic device-related infection and extraction trends in the U.S. Pacing Clin Electrophysiol 2017;40(3):286–93.

35. Kusumoto FM, Schoenfeld MH, Wilkoff BL, et al. 2017 HRS expert consensus statement on cardiovascular implantable electronic device lead management and extraction. Heart Rhythm 2017;14(12):e503–51.

36. Schaerf RHM, Najibi S, Conrad J. Percutaneous vacuum-assisted thrombectomy device used for removal of large vegetations on infected pacemaker and defibrillator leads as an adjunct to lead extraction. J Atr Fibrillation 2016;9(3):1455.

37. Patel N, Azemi T, Zaeem F, et al. Vacuum assisted vegetation extraction for the management of large lead vegetations. J Card Surg 2013;28(3):321–4.

38. Godara H, Jia KQ, Augostini RS, et al. Feasibility of concomitant vacuum-assisted removal of lead-related vegetations and cardiac implantable electronic device extraction. J Cardiovasc Electrophysiol 2018;29(10):1460–6.

39. Joseph-Alexis J, Jaffe A, Jacinto JP, et al. AngioVac removal of an isolated infected pulmonary valve papillary fibroelastoma. JACC Case Rep 2020;2(14):2213–6.

40. Bhagat A, Annie FH, Tager A, et al. Alternative treatment approach for right heart masses. Cureus 2018;10(12):e3673.

41. Qintar M, Wang DD, O'Neill WW, et al. Vacuum to the rescue: aspiration of a large mobile aortic arch thrombus with the AngioVac system utilizing transcaval access. J Invasive Cardiol 2021;33(9): E756–7.

42. Monastiriotis S, Gonzales C, Kokkosis A, et al. The use of AngioVac for symptomatic aortic thrombus complicated by mesenteric ischemia. Ann Vasc Surg 2016;32:129 e121–126.

43. Kang J, Fleischman F, Saremi F, et al. En bloc AngioVac removal of thoracic aortic mass. Tex Heart Inst J 2020;47(4):315–8.

44. Frisoli TM, So CY, Guruswamy JG, et al. Vacuuming in crowded dangerous spaces: aspiration of large ascending aortic thrombus. JACC Case Rep 2020; 2(12):1979–83.

45. Tsilimparis N, Spanos K, Debus ES, et al. Technical aspects of using the AngioVac system for thrombus aspiration from the ascending aorta. J Endovasc Ther 2018;25(5):550–3.

46. Ashukem M, Seibolt L, Verma DR, et al. A case of trans-septal left atrial thrombectomy utilizing AngioVac extracorporeal venous-venous cardiopulmonary bypass filter circuit in a patient with obstructive shock from large la and prosthetic valve thrombosis post tmvr. J Am Coll Cardiol 2019;73(9_ Supplement_1):1316.

47. Basman C, Rashid U, Parmar YJ, et al. The role of percutaneous vacuum-assisted thrombectomy for intracardiac and intravascular pathology. J Card Surg 2018;33(10):666–72.

Moving?

Make sure your subscription moves with you!

To notify us of your new address, find your **Clinics Account Number** (located on your mailing label above your name), and contact customer service at:

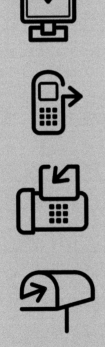

Email: journalscustomerservice-usa@elsevier.com

800-654-2452 (subscribers in the U.S. & Canada)
314-447-8871 (subscribers outside of the U.S. & Canada)

Fax number: 314-447-8029

Elsevier Health Sciences Division
Subscription Customer Service
3251 Riverport Lane
Maryland Heights, MO 63043

*To ensure uninterrupted delivery of your subscription, please notify us at least 4 weeks in advance of move.